T0291119

Living without Itch

A Johns Hopkins Press Health Book

LIVING
WITHOUT
ITCH

Proven Strategies and
Treatments for Relief

SECOND EDITION

Gil Yosipovitch, MD, and Zoe M. Lipman, MD

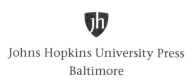

Johns Hopkins University Press
Baltimore

© 2025 Johns Hopkins University Press
All rights reserved. Published 2025
Printed in the United States of America on acid-free paper
9 8 7 6 5 4 3 2 1

Johns Hopkins University Press
2715 North Charles Street
Baltimore, Maryland 21218
www.press.jhu.edu

Library of Congress Cataloging-in-Publication Data is
available.

A catalog record for this book is available from the British
Library.

ISBN 978-1-4214-5045-2 (hardcover)
ISBN 978-1-4214-5046-9 (paperback)
ISBN 978-1-4214-5047-6 (ebook)

*Special discounts are available for bulk purchases of this book.
For more information, please contact Special Sales at
specialsales@jh.edu.*

Note to the Reader. This book is not meant to substitute for medical care of people with chronic itch, and treatment should not be based solely on its contents. Instead, treatment must be developed in a dialogue between the individual and their physician. Our book has been written to help with that dialogue.

Drug dosage: The author and publisher have made reasonable efforts to determine that the selection and dosage of drugs discussed in this text conform to the practices of the general medical community. The medications described do not necessarily have specific approval by the US Food and Drug Administration for use in the diseases and dosages for which they are recommended. In view of ongoing research, changes in governmental regulations, and the constant flow of information relating to drug therapy and drug reactions, the reader is urged to check the package insert of each drug for any change in indications and dosage and for warnings and precautions. This is particularly important when the recommended agent is a new and/or infrequently used drug.

Many of the images in this publication have been provided by VisualDx. VisualDx is a patient-specific diagnostic clinical decision support system and reference tool that links the benefits of conventional systems with high-quality images and proprietary problem-oriented search. More than 1,500 health care institutions rely on VisualDx to improve diagnostic accuracy, enhance medical education, and engage patients in their treatment and care.

One of the most challenging things for people with chronic itch is the sense of isolation. The feeling that there is no one else who is having the same experience. Individuals with chronic itch often report that itch interferes with their sleep and ability to engage in work, social, or recreational activities. Chronic itch has numerous causes, many of which are not well understood or effectively treated. In recent years, significant advancements in our understanding of mechanisms of itch and new treatments have been developed. This book follows our previous book *Living with Itch* (Johns Hopkins University Press, 2013) and provides useful information on different causes of itch and their management.

We hope this innovative book format that incorporates patients' perspectives will provide all people (patients, loved ones, and doctors) with helpful information on chronic itch and its management and empower patients in their care of this bothersome symptom.

I gratefully dedicate this book to the one in six people who suffer from chronic itch and continue to teach me daily lessons about itch. I also dedicate this book to my loving wife, Galit, and children, Natalie and Dan.

Gil Yosipovitch, MD

I would not be where I am today without the unconditional support of my parents, Marcy and Kenny, and younger sister, Kyra. I enthusiastically dedicate this book to them and all the patients who have inspired me with their strength and perseverance throughout my training.

Zoe M. Lipman, MD

Contents

Foreword

A Patient Perspective

My Story by Rachael Bronstein

At a young age, I needed to learn to be strong, resilient, and determined. My dad passed when he was 39 after a 10-year battle with a brain tumor. My mom was a teacher at the time, and my only sibling was my sister, who had special needs. My mom was amazing. She somehow kept it all together, raised us girls, and re-created herself. She became an independent financial planner and developed a very successful practice. I don't know if it was because I had to grow up quickly, or because I always wanted to do my best, but I was always determined.

In high school and college, I always tried to help people. I was a peer advisor, class president, and on the admissions team for prospective students. I volunteered at the Brain Tumor Society in Cambridge when I could. My dream was always to work at NBC, and after college, I was somehow able to make it happen. Shortly after starting this dream job, however, I started breaking out in a rash on my hands and eyelids—my first presentation of eczema, or atopic dermatitis. My mom attributed it to the stress of moving to a new city and job and often said that "happy stress" is sometimes just as much of a trigger as "unhappy stress." As I moved apartments often, met my husband, got married, and started having children, I did, indeed, experience a lot of happy stress.

When my first child was born, my eczema was OK. However, by my second child, it was awful. I was covered head to toe. I would cry when I had to shower and then immediately after would apply topical steroids and moisturizer everywhere and put on old clothes so new ones weren't ruined. It took up to two hours to find any relief!

The doctors didn't know what to do with me. We talked about more systemic treatments like cyclosporine and CellCept (mycophenolate mofetil), but there was a history of cancer in my family, and I was worried. Whether the worry was justified or not, I chose to suffer rather than suppress my immune system. The suffering was real and daily. The itching never stopped and the broken skin would get infected. One time, I ended up at my primary care doctor's office in town because my leg was so swollen that I could barely get my pants on. I needed to have intravenous antibiotics administered in the exam room, and if those failed, I would need to be admitted to the hospital for cellulitis. My husband would tell me to "stop itching," and I knew I needed to, but that was easier said than done.

On the treatment front, I felt as if I had tried everything. I found intermittent relief from using topical triamcinolone ointment and taking bleach baths, but I could never get cleared enough to do a consistent maintenance regimen. I tried seeing alternative medicine doctors to try steroid-free treatment alternatives. I even tried several extreme diets that were so restrictive they were impossible to follow long term while taking care of three young kids, working a full-time job, and continuing to manage my own skin. In fact, after eliminating dairy from my diet for so long, my body lost its ability to properly digest it and I eventually became allergic once it was reintroduced!

After my mom passed away from lung cancer in 2011 and my special needs sister was placed in a supportive care facility, I recognized stress to be an additional trigger of my scratching. I began to practice yoga and Pilates, go for daily walks, and sometimes just lay on my floor for 5–10 minutes and breathe to manage my stress. I grew acutely aware of both my known and potential triggers and did everything I could to eliminate them and set personal boundaries. I also began to keep an eczema journal, where I noted potential triggers, how much and what medications I was using, and how my eczema was doing so that I could evaluate and adjust as necessary. I self-motivated by telling myself that if my mom could juggle a sick husband, raise two kids (one of whom was special needs), and run her own business, then I could do this.

I had made significant strides in managing my eczema and knew exactly how to manage my flares when they occurred. However, each time I flared, I began to feel a little more depleted. After talking to Dr. Gil Yosipovitch, a world-renowned dermatologist who specializes in treating itch (and coauthor of this book!), I was ready to try something new. Dupilumab (i.e., Dupixent) was in its first year of Food and Drug Administration approval, and while I was initially reluctant to give it a shot, I am so glad that I eventually did. Within days of my first injection in December 2018, my flare on my hands started to clear and my itch significantly decreased. A few months later, my whole body was free of itch and rashes, and for the first time in so long, I was free of itch and the anxiety that came with it. While I know that dupilumab is not perfect and not for every person, it was an absolute game-changer for me.

Other than dupilumab, the most impactful factor in my eczema journey was learning about the National Eczema Association (NEA). I couldn't believe there was an entire organization and massive in-person expo dedicated to this condition that I had always tried to hide from others. I attended my first NEA expo in San Diego in 2009 and have since been to seven others! It is truly an incredible experience to learn from experts, take workshops, learn about the most recent advancements in the management of our condition, and network with others suffering from the same disease. In fact, I am so passionate about the NEA and their dedication to improving the lives of those suffering from eczema that I have sat on the Board of Directors for the past three years. In addition to the NEA, there are many regional, local, and even virtual support groups and educational programs to help support you on your journey.

In the past three years, I have remained on dupilumab and have not required any antibiotics, oral or topical steroids, or bleach baths. On occasion, I have had a facial flare, and I have treated it with topical tacrolimus (Protopic). I still practice self-care, take daily walks, and set boundaries when facing stressful situations. I do have trouble with the heat, but as long as I take along a wet towel with me, I can enjoy outdoors activities. I was even able to go to Greece for the first time this summer! I would never have considered it before due to the heat and sweat, which would have exacerbated my eczema. I also spent this year figuring out what makes me happy professionally and I launched a new company.

My itch journey, like many others, has been long and painful, but I do believe there are enough tools in our large itch toolkits for everyone to find improvement. While some of the things I tried did not fix my skin, I eventually found the routines and practices that worked for me. The purpose of this book is to educate you, empower you, and equip you with the knowledge to advocate for yourself and find relief from the monster that is itch.

I would like to dedicate this to my mother, my cheerleader and role model, my incredible husband, Ronnie, who stood by my side through it all, and my loving children, Ben, Jeremy, and Rebecca. Special thanks to Dr. Yosipovitch and the amazing people and community that make up the National Eczema Association. You are a true gift.

Online Supplement

Living without Itch, Second Edition, is supported by an online supplement. It provides color versions of the images in the book as well as animated videos illustrating the conditions and techniques discussed by the authors. The additional materials for this book can be found by visiting the specific book page on press.jhu.edu.

Living without Itch

1. Introduction to Itch

1.1 What Is Itch?

Itch is a symptom that we've all experienced at some point in our lives. Whether it be from a bug bite, an uncomfortable fabric in our clothing, or a new rash that appeared, we can all describe the feeling of having a strong desire to scratch our skin and obtain immediate relief. This intense feeling we call "itch" was first described in 1660 by German physician Samuel Hafenreffer, who defined itch as "an unpleasant sensation provoking the desire to scratch." But while itch is something we can all relate to, some people experience it more frequently and intensely than others.

The list of potential reasons why we itch at any particular moment is enormous. To narrow down this list, we must accurately categorize and describe the itch that is being experienced. The first way to do this is through its duration.

Acute itch is a sensation that causes the urge to scratch for a limited time, ranging anywhere from a few seconds to six weeks. This itch can result from an insect bite (like a mosquito bite), an exposure to a plant (like poison ivy), an illness (like chickenpox), or even an irritation (like wearing an itchy fabric or having dry skin). Whatever the cause, acute itch is typically limited to the affected area(s), where you may notice swelling (inflammation) and/or redness (erythema). Acute itch can usually be treated successfully with antihistamines or steroid creams that can be purchased over-the-counter or prescribed by your doctor.

Chronic itch is itch lasting longer than six weeks. If you are reading this book, it is likely that you or someone you love is suffering from this type, and therefore, this will be our main focus. Chronic itch, as opposed to acute itch, usually originates from within the body rather than outside of it. A long list of complex medical problems can produce itch and may also affect a number of other organs within the body. These include not only skin diseases but also systemic diseases, neurologic diseases, and psychiatric disorders. In addition, chronic itch may result from long-term exposure to irritating external agents like nickel or poison ivy.

Chronically itchy conditions are usually harder to treat than acutely itchy conditions, as traditional treatments such as antihistamines (like Benadryl, Zyrtec, and Claritin) often do not provide long-term, if any, relief. This is because these treatment methods typically do not target the root cause of the itch-causing disease. **Intractable itch** is a term used to describe a chronic itch that has not been relieved after multiple treatment attempts. Luckily, in the past decade, we have advanced our understanding about mechanisms and causes of itch. As we continue to learn more about *why* we itch, we also find more, and better, options for treatment. Because of this, living *without* itch (specifically, chronic itch) is a greater possibility than ever before.

1.2 How Many People Itch? (Epidemiology)

While everyone has experienced the sensation of itch at one point or another, some people encounter it more frequently and intensely than others. Recent estimates show that about one in five people (~22%) throughout the world experience chronic itch at some point in their life. Additionally, 25% of people with chronic itch state that they've suffered from itch for more than five years. It is also known that the prevalence of itch tends to increase with age, particularly in those older than 65 years.

As we stated above, chronic itch can develop in a wide variety of dermatologic, systemic, and neurologic conditions. Table 1.1 and table 1.2 show the prevalence of itch in a selected subset of these conditions.

1.3 Why Do I Itch? (Mechanisms)

Basic Skin Structure

To understand why we itch, it is important to first understand the basic structure of our skin and how these structures communicate with our brain and motor system (behaviors).

Table 1.1 Estimated Itch Cases Prevalence Rate for Selected Skin Disorders

Dermatologic condition	Prevalence rate (%)
Atopic dermatitis	100
Scabies	100
Prurigo nodularis	89
Urticaria (hives)	76
Psoriasis	70
Burns	67–87
Dry skin associated with old age	30–60

Table 1.2 Estimated Itch Prevalence Rate for Selected Systemic Diseases

Systemic disease	Prevalence rate (%)
Chronic renal failure (on hemodialysis)	55–85
Hyperthyroidism	60
Anorexia nervosa	58
Polycythemia vera	48
Chronic liver disease	40
Hodgkin's lymphoma	30
HIV (on antiretroviral therapy)	31
Diabetes	11
Leukemia	5
Other malignancy	2–26

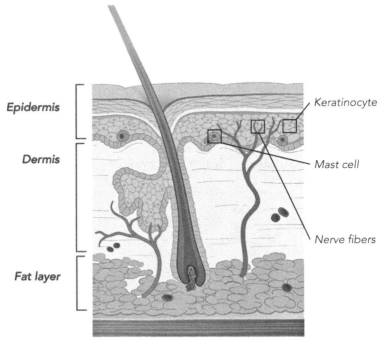

Figure 1.1 Basic structures of the skin. Author photo.

The main function of our skin is to provide our internal organs with a barrier to the outside world, providing protection from infection, physical injury, and ultraviolet rays, as well as preventing moisture, heat, and water loss. In addition, our skin is also a sensory organ, headlined by our sense of "touch" and our ability to sense different temperatures, pressures, pain, and itch. The structure of the skin reflects these functions.

The skin has several layers that all work together to carry out the above functions. The top layer of the skin, called the *epidermis*, contains most of the cells that produce color pigment (*melanocytes* that produce *melanin*) that make your skin the color it is, shielding you from the sun's harmful UV rays; it also is your main barrier to the outside world, protecting you from disease and trauma and water loss. Underneath the epidermis is the *dermis*, which contains your oil and sweat glands as well as fibrous and elastic tissues. Your hair follicles also originate here. Further down beneath the dermis is your subcutaneous tissue, which contains your fat cells and large blood vessels.

Transmission of Itch by Nerves

The nerves that allow you to sense itch on your skin originate in your epidermis and run all the way through the dermis, subcutaneous tissue, and spinal cord. Most of these nerves, called *C fibers*, are a subset of nerves that have a very slow conduction speed (only 2 to 8 cm/s). When C fibers in the skin detect something "itchy," they transmit this sensation to the *dorsal root ganglion*: an area right outside of the spinal cord where these C fibers can

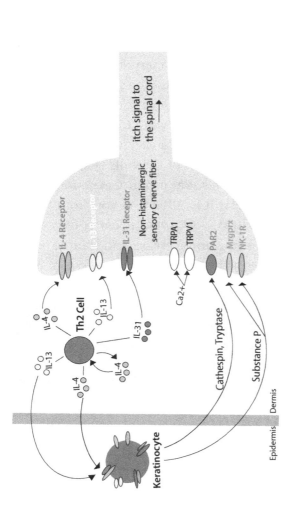

Figure 1.2 Some of the many substances and receptors involved in itch transmission from the skin to the brain within the nonhistaminergic pathway. *Cytokines*, including **interleukins (ILs)** and **thymic stromal lymphoprotein (TSLP)**, are part of the immune system. **Cathepsin** and **tryptase** are enzymes that break down proteins, otherwise known as proteases. Substance P is a first indicated in pain but has also been found to be involved in itch transmission. Each of these compounds binds to a specific receptor on the neuron. **Transient receptor potential (TRP)** channels are a unique type of receptor on the neuron that is activated by temperature changes. Author photo.

synapse (communicate) with the nerves that will bring
the signal up to the brain. The neurons that carry the
itch signal to the brain are part of the *lateral spinothalamic
tract*—one of many tracts that bring signals up and down
the spinal cord and connect the brain with the rest of
your body.

Do You Want to Learn More?

See online supplement for an interactive graphic on
the itch pathway from the skin to the brain.

Once in the brain, these itch signals are processed and
organized in the *thalamus* and "forwarded" to different
brain areas that allow you to recognize that you feel itchy,
emotionally process the itch, and initiate scratching
behaviors.

So What Causes an "Itchy Sensation"?

Many compounds and chemicals within the skin can
cause your C fibers to begin transmitting itch signals
toward the brain. In fact, numerous substances can induce
itch in different diseases and disorders; researchers have
prioritized understanding of these substances so that we
can better treat itchy diseases. In its most basic sense,
these substances can be divided into *histaminergic* and
nonhistaminergic.

Histamine-triggered itch: The term "histaminergic"
refers to a pathway that involves the chemical histamine:
an important immune system chemical that is released from

mast cells and triggers an immune response. Depending on the amount of histamine that is released, this immune response can produce localized or generalized swelling (edema) and redness (erythema). Examples of "histaminergic" itch include hives (urticaria), insect bites, and drug rashes. It's because of this mechanism that commonly used drugs like antihistamines can often successfully resolve itch in these conditions.

Nonhistaminergic itch: While antihistamines may be the first drug you reach for when you feel itchy, it is unlikely to help with most chronic itchy conditions. That's because most itchy conditions do not act through a histaminergic pathway. A number of immune system compounds and chemicals fall within this nonhistaminergic umbrella, many of which we are still researching and trying to understand. Some examples include cytokines (components of the immune system), opioids (the same category of compounds we use for pain relief), bile acids (produced by your liver), and proteases (enzymes that break down proteins). We will talk about these in more detail when we discuss the new targeted treatments that are available or in development for itch.

Itch and Pain

There are many similarities between chronic itch and chronic pain, starting with the C nerve fibers that use the same lateral spinothalamic tract in the spine to bring sensory signals from the skin up to the brain. In both conditions, overactivation (*hypersensitization*) of nerve fibers also can cause stimuli to be perceived as increasingly itchy or painful. For example, in chronically itchy people, a typically painful stimulus (such as an electric shock) may actually be interpreted as itchy, whereas in a patients with chronic pain, an itchy fabric may actually aggravate pain. In addition, both conditions have been shown to be terribly bothersome to patients, have a large impact on quality of life, and be difficult to treat, but there are also some key differences between the two.

When you encounter something that is painful, such as touching a hot stove or stepping on a piece of glass, your instinctual reaction is to immediately pull your hand or foot away from the area where the pain was caused. When you feel itchy, however, your instinctual response is to scratch the area and, in turn, touch it. What do these two different responses have to do with each other? Ever scratched so hard you began to bleed? Turns out, the pain caused by scratching an itch might actually inhibit the sensation of itch. In fact, many therapies we recommend for chronic itch act through this mechanism, such as capsaicin cream (the active ingredient in hot chili peppers!) and very hot or cold showers.

You might be thinking, if increasing pain decreases itch, does decreasing pain increase itch? In some ways, yes! For example, patients with postoperative or chronic pain taking opioid drugs (think: morphine or oxycodone) for pain relief have been shown to have increased itch—however, research has also shown that this is not solely due to the decrease in pain but rather the dual function of a subtype of opioid receptor (the mu-opioid receptor) that, when activated, decreases pain but can induce itch.

1.4 Terminology in Dermatology

Throughout the book, we may use terms that may be used colloquially but have more specific definitions when referring to skin diseases. The following is a list of useful definitions to help you get the most out of this book:

General Terminology

Lesion: Any single area of altered skin; may be singular or multiple.

Rash: A widespread eruption of lesions.

Dermatosis: Generic term used to describe a disease of the skin.

Lesion Morphology (Structure/Appearance)

Macule: A small, flat area of skin that is altered in color.

Patch: A larger flat area of skin that is altered in color.

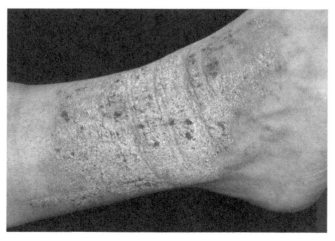

Figure 1.3 **Lichen simplex chronicus** is a disease characterized by local lichenification, which involves thickening of the skin as a result of repetitive scratching. Areas commonly affected include the wrists, ankles, back, and genitals. Author photo.

Papule: A small, elevated lesion.

Nodule: A larger elevated lesion.

Plaque: An elevated lesion with well-defined borders.

Vesicle: A small blister.

Bulla: A large blister.

Pustule: A papule filled with pus.

Wheal: An acute elevation of skin due to edema, often pale in the center and red/pink further out.

Secondary Skin Changes

Lichenification: Caused by chronic rubbing, which results in palpably thickened skin.

Crusting: The result of fluid seeping through and drying on top of eroded skin.

Excoriation: A loss of the epidermis and a portion of the dermis due to scratching or other external injury. It may be linear or punctate.

Erosion: A sore due to the superficial or partial destruction of surface tissue such as the skin.

Fissure: A split, crack, erosion or narrow ulceration of the skin.

Ulcer: The full-thickness loss of the epidermis plus at least a portion of the dermis; it may extend into the subcutaneous tissue. An ulcer heals with a scar.

Hypertrophy: When some component of the skin is enlarged or has grown excessively.

Prurigo nodule: A firm dome-shaped, smooth-topped, or crusted nodule that forms secondary to chronic scratching.

2. Understanding My Itch

In this chapter, we will go through some of the most common conditions that cause both acute and chronic itch.

2.1 Acute Itch

2.1.1 Insect Bites

All of us have experienced the pesky itch (pun intended) of a bug bite at some point in our lifetime. When an insect, such as a mosquito, bites you, it pierces your skin to suck up blood; in the process, its saliva makes its way into your skin. Your body's immune system recognizes this saliva as a foreign substance and attacks it, causing blood filled with immune cells to rush to the area (inflammation). This results in swelling as well as the itchiness you experience, and the size of your "bite bump" represents how strongly your immune system reacts. You may react more strongly to a bug bite if you have a disorder causing your immune system to be more reactive or are bitten by a species your body previously developed an immune response to. While insect bites are typically self-limited, meaning they will resolve on their own over the course of a few hours to days, the itch experienced while waiting for that to occur can be extremely bothersome. You can decrease this itch by using an ice pack to reduce swelling and temporarily numb the area or by applying a topical antihistamine or anti-inflammatory cream.

Did You Know?

People who think that they get bitten by mosquitos more frequently than others often refer to themselves as having "sweet skin." And while they might not necessarily have more sugar in their blood or skin, there is some truth to this. Studies have shown that your genetics can play a role in how "attractive" you are to mosquitos. Some of these genes contribute to body odor. In addition, females have been reported to experience greater itch in response to mosquito bites than males.

2.1.2 Acute Urticaria (Hives)

Urticaria is another word for hives, which are red, typically very itchy, raised bumps of the skin. These elevated lesions can come and go over a period of only a few hours and often appear as a result of contact with an allergen or irritant, such as a specific ingredient in food, soaps, or detergents or an environmental trigger. The cause of these lesions is the release of a chemical called **histamine** and other inflammatory substances by **mast cells**, a type of white blood cell (a concept referred to as *degranulation*). Histamine binds to specific **receptors** near the skin, subsequently causing inflammation (swelling and redness) in the surrounding skin areas. Sometimes, a

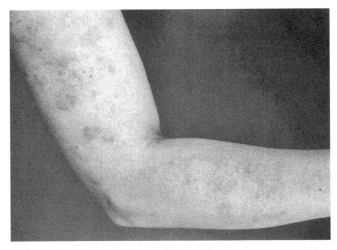

Figure 2.1 Acute urticaria or "hives." Image appears with permission from VisualDx © Logical Images, Inc.

triggering substance can easily be identified, and so, removal/avoidance of that substance can be a useful measure in treatment and future prevention. In addition, antihistamines can be used to block histamine binding to its receptor, preventing further and future inflammation.

2.1.3 Acute Contact Dermatitis

Contact dermatitis refers to any rash that arises from contact of the skin with a substance and has two sub-types: (1) allergic, in which contact with a substance triggers an immune response that damages the skin, and (2) irritant, in which a substance directly irritates and damages the skin. It typically results in a red-colored rash with sharp borders that outline areas of the skin that

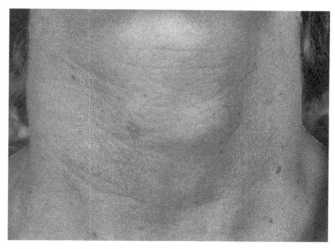

Figure 2.2 An allergic contact dermatitis reaction to nickel, a common component of fashion jewelry and one of the most common allergens. Image appears with permission from VisualDx © Logical Images, Inc.

were in contact with the triggering substance or material. The rash typically presents two to seven days after exposure to the trigger and can persist until the triggering substance is identified and removed—as such, classification as acute or chronic itch depends on how quickly the trigger is identified and eliminated. Additionally, some patients may experience what we call an "id reaction"— that is, a rash that develops in a body area different from the site of contact with a trigger due to a secondary immune response. Common triggers include new cosmetics or creams (especially fragranced ones), metals (fashion jewelry, nickel), occupational exposures, and exposure to plants (poison ivy).

2.2 Chronic Itch

2.2.1 Xerosis (Dry Skin)

Xerosis, or dry skin, can occur at any age. It is one of the most common skin conditions in the middle-aged and elderly population and has a prevalence estimated to be

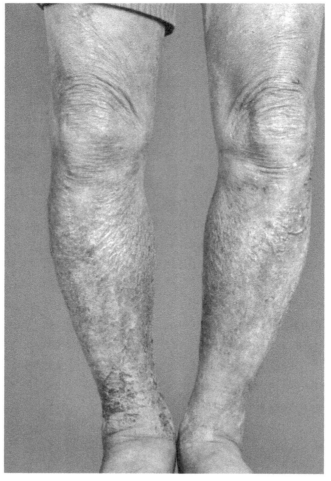

Figure 2.3 Severe xerosis (dry skin). Author photo.

anywhere between 29% and 85% of these age groups. Xerosis can present in different ways that range in visibility from obvious to extremely subtle, as well as localized to specific areas or generalized across the entire body. It usually presents with skin scaling, roughness, and/or cracks (fissures) and can be associated with feelings of itching, burning, skin "tightness," or pain. The most common triggers of dry skin include environmental factors (cold, low humidity/dry indoor heat [commonly described as *winter itch*], or intense sunlight exposure) and skin cleansing/washing (long/hot showers, alkaline [high pH] soaps, and cleansing agents). If identified, xerosis is treated by avoiding triggers and using topical emollients (moisturizers). However, generalized xerosis may also present secondary to other conditions like systemic diseases or may be drug induced.

2.2.2 Inflammatory Skin Conditions

Atopic Dermatitis (Eczema)

Atopic dermatitis (AD), known more commonly as "eczema," is a chronic skin disorder that affects hundreds of millions of people worldwide and is continuing to increase in prevalence. It can affect persons of any age but most frequently affects young children. It is characterized by periodic flares of dry, flakey, and inflamed skin, which, through scratching, can lead to redness, crusting, scaling, and oozing. AD lesions develop in typical distributions that often include the skin folds of the arms, behind the knees, and below the ears. However, the hallmark of AD is the intense itch it causes.

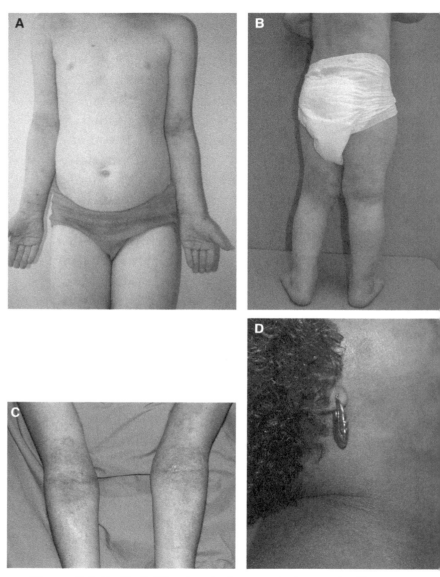

Figure 2.4 (A, B, C, D) Atopic dermatitis (eczema) affecting the skin folds in children (A, B) and adults (C, D). Images A and B courtesy of Dr. Elaine C. Siegfried. Images C and D appear with permission from VisualDx © Logical Images, Inc.

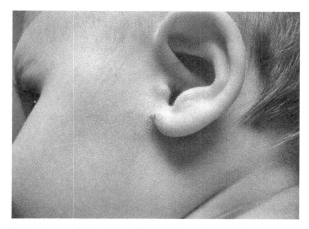

Figure 2.5 A crack in the skin below the earlobe, known as an *infra-auricular fissure*, is often associated with severe atopic dermatitis. Author photo.

What Causes AD? Unfortunately, there is no short answer to the question, "What causes atopic dermatitis?" The mechanism behind AD and its associated itch is multifactorial and involves complex interactions between the immune system, the external environment, and one's genetics. In recent years, our understanding of how these domains interact with one another has expanded greatly; however, we still have a long way to go. Here we will discuss our most up-to-date knowledge on the cause of AD.

Role of the Immune System in AD Part of what is known as the "allergic triad" alongside asthma and seasonal allergies (hay fever), AD has been shown to be caused by an overactive immune system. We know that cytokines, substances produced by immune cells that are used to activate more immune cells and nerves, are often present in greater numbers in people with AD—this results in a downhill cascade of events that eventually leads to the visible symptoms you see on the skin.

Do You Want to Learn More?

See online supplement for an interactive graphic on how the hypersensitivity of nerve fibers causes itch in atopic dermatitis (eczema).

Type 2 T cells, a subtype of white blood cells, are particularly involved in this process by migrating into the skin and secreting cytokines to trigger atopic dermatitis. Many of the newer treatments for AD ("biologics") target these cytokines and this cascade of events, aiming to stop its progression at different points. But what triggers the immune system to activate and produce these cytokines? The answer lies somewhere between your genetics and your environment.

Role of Genetics in AD There is no single "AD gene" that can be passed down through generations and causes you to develop the disease; however, we do know of multiple genes that may increase your susceptibility to environmental triggers and make you more likely to develop AD. One of these genes codes for a protein named *filaggrin*—one of the proteins that makes up the **stratum corneum**, the most upper layer of the epidermis. A variant in filaggrin weakens the skin barrier, making it more penetrable to germs, allergens, and other foreign substances, all of which may trigger the immune system to react and irritate nerve fibers. In addition, such genetic variants may also impact the skin barrier by leading to increased water loss and resulting in the dry skin that those with AD experience.

Did You Know?

As we have many new technologies and companies now that can help you explore your own genetics, you might be wondering if you should try and identify which genes you have or if your loved ones are "at risk." Our opinion: save your money. The role of many suspected genes in AD is still very unclear. In addition, simply having a defect in one or many of these genes does not guarantee that AD will develop.

In addition to filaggrin, many other genes have been recently identified that may have implications in producing AD. Other genes that code for compounds involved in skin structure have been shown to be *downregulated* (produce less of the compound they code for), while genes that code for aspects of the immune system have been shown to be *upregulated* (produce more of the compound they code for). Any combination of genes that produces defects in the skin barrier and/or increases the immune response can make you more susceptible to developing AD.

The Environment and AD Your genetics can increase your susceptibility and reactivity to environmental triggers. So, if you eliminate triggers, AD won't develop, right? Not so fast. While some people with AD notice specific triggers, such as temperatures, foods, or personal care products/ingredients that aggravate their AD, many others have a difficult time identifying such factors. Allergen patch testing can be used to identify specific allergens that may irritate your skin; however, the relationship between allergens identified in this manner and what actually impacts the development and severity of AD cannot be determined (Are these allergens actually triggering AD, or is the overactive AD immune system increasing reactivity to these allergens?). Moreover, many of the environmental triggers of AD may be out of your control. The increasing global prevalence of AD cannot be explained by genetics alone, and factors such as climate change, pollution, and even improved hygiene have been suggested as possible factors contributing to this increase. And yes, you read that right—being "too clean" may not be that great for you (at least in the case of AD).

Did You Know?

Winter itch is a form of eczema in adults that is characterized by the skin becoming abnormally dry, itchy, and cracked during the winter months. The lower legs and forearms tend to be especially affected. The treatment for winter itch is to regularly apply moisturizers and topical corticosteroid ointments.

Did You Know?

People who live in urban areas and regions with low humidity have an increased risk of developing AD.

Itch in AD Itch is the most common symptom experienced by patients with AD and also one of the most debilitating. Severe and frequent itch has been shown to impact patients' sleep, mood, and overall quality of life. It also contributes to many psychosocial conditions, including depression, anxiety, concentration difficulties, and poor self-esteem. The itch experienced in AD may be caused by a combination of both skin dryness and inflammation. It can also be aggravated by proteases (enzymes that break down proteins) produced by dust mites or *Staphylococcus aureus* bacteria, a natural inhabitant of the skin and respiratory tract or proteases secreted by immune and skin cells. While scratching may cause immediate relief, it may actually worsen the itch in the long term by trapping you within the "itch–scratch cycle." The more you itch, the more you scratch, the more damage you do to your skin barrier, and more environmental compounds can penetrate and irritate the skin, causing more itching and scratching.

While itch in AD may stress you out, stress itself may also induce or aggravate itch. Brain imaging studies have shown that itch in AD activates brain areas involved in emotion and memory of negative experiences.

Fully managing itch in AD requires managing all the components described above that may induce or aggravate itch, including inflammation, exposure to environmental triggers and allergens, emotional stress, and infections (see table 2.1). In addition, it often requires significant efforts by a patient's support system to avoid triggers and assist with treatments. As such, comprehensive treatment for AD itch should be targeted for the age and circumstances of the individual and include both preventative and reactionary

Table 2.1 Common Triggers of Itch in People Who Have Atopic Dermatitis

Environmental factors	Low and high humidity Cold and hot weather Seasonal allergies
Allergens and irritants	Harsh soaps and detergents Food (peanuts and seafood are frequent offenders) Pets (cat and dog dander) Mite exposure Wool Perfumes Cigarette smoke
Stress	Includes emotional factors such as divorce, loss of a loved one, work, school, or other significant life changes
Infections	The most common skin infection is *Staphylococcus aureus*

measures for active itch. You can read more about such treatments in chapter 3 of this book!

My Experience with Atopic Dermatitis

By Kyle Bruner

My name is Kyle Bruner and I am a nineteen-year-old eczema warrior from Ontario, Canada. I was diagnosed with atopic dermatitis in infancy, and by the time I was one year old, I was suffering with severe eczema that required several hospital and doctors' appointments each week.

My earliest memories of my life with itch are of me being wrapped in bandages and towels to keep me from scratching and bleeding. My parents talked to me about how they had to dress me in backward sleepers and taped gloves on my hands, but I would chew through them until I bled because the itch was so bad. My doctors had me on multiple oral antibiotics, topical creams and lotions, oral painkillers, and antihistamines and still nothing helped.

My eczema was the severe trifecta, which included anaphylaxis and asthma. My IgE, a type of immunoglobulin or antibody that is activated in allergic processes, was high. In fact, my IgE levels were so high that the doctors kept testing because they thought it was an error. Living with eczema is like being on a roller coaster ride for the first time—you have no idea which way it will go on any given day and the triggers change constantly too. The effects on my mental health were so bad—I got to a point where I didn't think I could endure another day of it. When you are living with a disease like this, it isn't always visible to those around you, but it is always there and relentlessly affecting every choice, every thought, and everything you do. Do you try to go to the sleepover where you will be up all night itching? Should you try to go on the camping trip where I could flare without AC or have an allergy attack? Can I go to the high school where they have a uniform that is polyester?

As I entered high school, my journey got really dark and I almost didn't make it through due to the stress, bullying, and lack of sleep. Kids at school made fun of me and called me names and my vice principal would harass me about my skin—itching in my mandated uniform was not allowed, even while knowing that certain clothes would make me irritated with this condition. When I went to see the vice principal during a very bad flare, she told me to get over it and asked me what I wanted her to do about it. My parents pulled me out of that school and searched for help.

We found the National Eczema Association and the Eczema Society of Canada, and suddenly there was a light at the end of the tunnel. We found a community where I not only fit in but thrived. I was lucky to have met Dr. Richard Aron and Dr. Peter Lio, who have guided me since on my eczema journey, which I am happy to say is much happier and more promising than ever.

The best advice I would give to someone suffering with eczema is that it truly is an uphill battle. Some days you just won't win, but that's OK. Living with my eczema, and fighting these battles daily, I've learned not to let them define me. Instead, I use each challenge and backward step to grow and adapt so that next time I face that same battle, I'm more prepared than before. If you're suffering from eczema, I encourage you to keep fighting and believe that you will overcome. Listen to your doctors, find those who support and understand you, leave situations that cause more harm than good, and practice mindfulness to help you push through the pain and difficult times—I promise, it will get better.

Other Eczematous Skin Diseases
Several other itchy skin diseases share similar mechanisms and/or have similar rashes to atopic dermatitis.

These conditions include contact dermatitis, dyshidrotic eczema (palmoplantar dermatitis), seborrheic dermatitis, nummular eczema, and stasis dermatitis.

In section 2.2.3, we discussed **contact dermatitis** in the acute setting. However, if the triggering substance or environmental factor is not quickly identified and avoided or removed, this condition may become chronic. For this reason, if you suspect a contact reaction, it is important to determine the offending agent, whether that be through trial and error or patch testing.

Dyshidrotic eczema is a chronic recurrence of blisters on the palms and/or soles that is extremely itchy. It is most frequently found on the sides and palm side of the fingers. These blisters are often said to resemble tapioca pudding. This condition may worsen or be first noticed after excessive handwashing or hand sanitizer usage. It

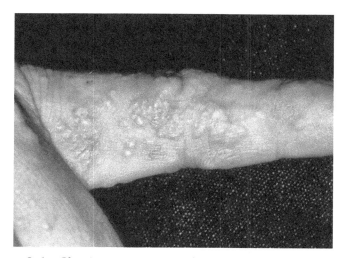

Figure 2.6 Classic presentation of dyshidrotic eczema with tiny "tapioca-like" vesicles on the side of the finger. Image appears with permission from VisualDx © Logical Images, Inc.

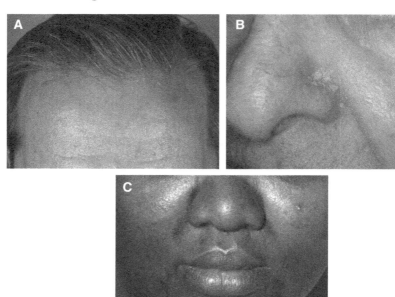

Figure 2.7 (A, B, C) Seborrheic dermatitis of the scalp (A), nasolabial fold (B, C), and chin (C). Images appear with permission from VisualDx © Logical Images, Inc.

could be related to allergic responses, and emotional stress can both trigger and aggravate it.

Seborrheic dermatitis is an extremely common skin disorder that can occur throughout the life span (often referred to as "cradle cap" in infants, "dandruff" in adults when mild and on the scalp). It appears as areas of redness with overlying yellow, greasy-looking scales and is most commonly seen on the scalp, center of the face, external ear, upper trunk, and groin area. Its presence has been correlated with the presence of *Malassezia*, a fungus, as well as stress.

Psoriasis

Psoriasis is another common chronic skin condition that affects about 3% of the US adult population, including more than 7.5 million individuals. It consists of thick, raised red lesions with a silvery-white scaly top layer. While these lesions can appear on any area of the body, they most frequently appear on the scalp, elbows, knees, trunk, and genital regions. The most common form of psoriasis is **plaque** psoriasis, which typically fits the description above. However, other forms of psoriasis include **erythrodermic** (severe redness spanning a large surface area), **guttate** (smaller red spots appearing together on the skin), **pustular** (white blisters with pus surrounded by areas of redness), and **inverse** (skin redness occurs in body folds such as the groin and armpits) psoriasis. In all forms of psoriasis, itch is an extremely common and bothersome symptom. In fact, the term "psoriasis" comes from the Latin word "psora," meaning itch.

Cause of Psoriasis Psoriasis is considered an autoimmune condition, which means that the body's own immune system attacks healthy skin. In doing so, the skin's cell production process is sped up faster than the rate at which dead skin cells naturally "fall off," resulting in an excess growth of skin cells and the formation of those raised, scaly plaques. The typical life cycle of a skin cell is around one month, but in psoriasis, this entire process lasts only a few days. Most treatments for psoriasis lesions involve decreasing the activity of the immune system, with newer, more targeted treatments ("biologics")

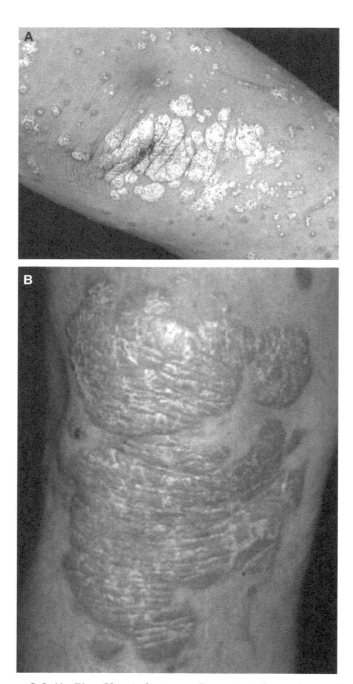

Figure 2.8 (A, B) Classic lesions of psoriasis featuring scaly, flaky, white plaques on the elbows (A) and knees (B). Image A appears with permission from VisualDx © Logical Images, Inc. Image B is from the collection of the authors.

targeting psoriasis-specific points within the immune cascade.

Psoriatic Itch Most people who suffer from psoriasis are affected by itch in some form, whether it be generalized throughout many parts of the body or localized to specific areas such as the scalp. The desire to scratch is particularly important in psoriasis because it not only can lead to perpetuation of the itch–scratch cycle but also may increase the development of future skin lesions. The appearance of psoriatic lesions in areas of trauma, such as scratching, is known as the *Koebner phenomenon*. The scalp is one of the most commonly itchy sites in psoriasis.

While the specific cause of itch in psoriasis is still not fully understood, it likely involves components of both the immune and neurologic systems. Many treatments for psoriatic lesions that target the body's immune system can improve itch, often before the skin lesions themselves improve. In addition, treatments that target the nerves can decrease the sensation of itch in many patients. These will be discussed in detail in chapter 3.

My Experience with Psoriasis

By Chip Newton

I have always been a very tough and resilient person. As a college baseball player, you kind of have to be that way. Working through the hitting slumps, waking up at the crack of dawn, and cramming for that economics exam when you're exhausted from a full day of practice—challenges are a part of the daily routine, and persevering was in my nature.

After graduating from college, moving to New York City, and working at my dream job, my confidence was at an all-time high. That is, until I noticed chunks of my hair falling out. Like all challenges before, I confronted this one head-on by seeing a dermatologist right away. I was diagnosed with seborrheic dermatitis, given a prescription shampoo, and thought my problem was solved. But my hair continued to fall out, my scalp became progressively itchier, and I quickly realized this misdiagnosis was only the beginning of the challenges I would soon face.

When I moved across the country to California for graduate school, my itch came with me. Within weeks of the move, I scheduled an appointment with a new dermatologist who diagnosed me with psoriasis. I was promptly referred to a specialty pharmacy that prepared coal tar solutions to rub on my scalp, but the relief was minimal. I started to flake, and the itch started to spread nearly everywhere on my body—my back, trunk, elbows, knees, fingers, and toes all began to itch and flake constantly with little relief. Having the proper diagnosis was helpful, but at the time over 30 years ago, there weren't many great treatment options available. Luckily, within those past 30 years, that has changed.

Now, at the age of 57, I look back on my time dealing with my psoriasis diagnosis impressed with the progress that has been made within the field of medicine, but even more impressed with my own resilience and determination to overcome challenge after challenge. As Babe Ruth famously once said, "Don't let the fear of striking out keep you from playing the game"; in my case, the fear was trying another failed treatment, and the game was preventing my psoriasis from ruining my life. Between body soaks, UV light therapy, synthetic vitamin D, steroids, and immunosuppressants, I tried every new treatment as it became available. Some provided more relief than others, some for longer than others, but eventually the itch and flaking always returned. Once confident showing off my athletic build at the beach and gym, I started wearing long-sleeve shirts to hide my disease. When no one was looking, I would scratch my back against my office door. I lost lots of sleep. The constant presence of itch and flaking almost brought me to my knees several times, but the strong desire to reach my end goal kept motivating me to try new things. Giving up was never an option.

For me, monoclonal antibody therapy was the savior I was waiting for, first secukinumab (Cosentyx), then guselkumab (Tremfya). These therapies were able to control my itch, and for the first time I can remember, actually forget about itch for prolonged periods of time. Today, on guselkumab, is the best that I've ever felt in 35 years (other than the few extra pounds I've put on . . .).

Throughout all of the trials and tribulations of living with my psoriasis and itch, there were several constants that got me through the worst. The first was distraction—using any type of activity, work, exercise, and so on to distract me from my itching. The second was my mom's old bathing cap, which I slept with to occlude my prescribed scalp solution and helped to prevent itching and bleeding and loosened up my psoriatic plaques. However, the single most important factor in my journey was the constant and nonjudgmental support of my now wife who kept me laughing, motivated, and confident through it all. From helping me explain to others at the pool that psoriasis is not contagious, to taking silly pictures of me in my tar bath and laughing with me about them, to exhibiting true patience and empathy when I was at my lowest points.

If there is any advice I can give to others going through the same things, it would be to not let your disease define you—maintain your confidence and positive outlook, and rely on your support system when you find yourself struggling. With perseverance, strength, and a little help from some really smart doctors and scientists, living life without constant itch is possible.

Prurigo Nodularis

Prurigo nodularis (PN) is an extremely itchy skin condition in which hard, crusty bumps form on the skin. These lesions are naturally skin colored and dry with a rough texture but are often red and scabbed due to the frequent and hard scratching that occurs. Scars formed from old lesions are typically white. PN usually appears in areas that are easy to reach and scratch, such as the arms, shoulders, and legs. Someone with PN may have only a few lesions or dozens. These lesions are typically the end result of persistent and intense scratching. The initial itch-causing trigger can differ from person to person and, in many cases, is never identified. However, while difficult, treatment of PN itch is still possible using some of

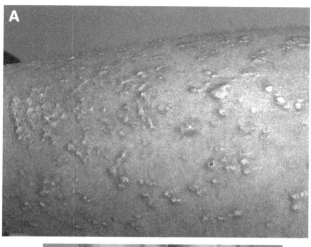

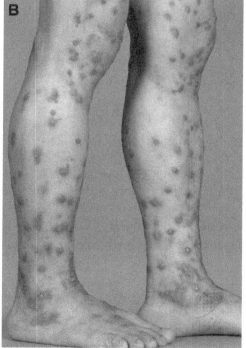

Figure 2.9 (A, B) Prurigo nodularis. Image A appears with permission from VisualDx © Logical Images, Inc. Image B is from the collection of the authors.

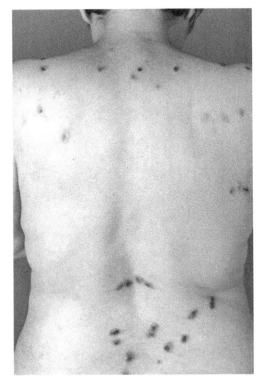

Figure 2.10 The **butterfly sign** appears in skin rashes that are caused directly by the act of scratching. The area in the center of the back that is difficult to reach and scratch is typically spared and roughly resembles a butterfly. Author photo.

the therapies that target the immune system and itch-transmitting nerves discussed later in this book.

My Experience with Prurigo Nodularis

By David Baker

Itch was never an issue in my life. Sure, I had the occasional bothersome mosquito bite or hive here and there, but nothing antihistamines, some distraction, and a little time couldn't fix. That is, until four years ago, at the age of 53, when I suddenly woke up one day with intense itching all over my body that didn't go away.

At the time, I was at a juncture in my professional life and experiencing a ton of stress, but I had been stressed before and it certainly was never accompanied by itching. Could it have been bed bugs from the hotel I recently stayed at? Was I newly allergic to something? Was there something wrong with my internal organs? It appeared so suddenly, out of the blue, and just continued getting worse. I needed to find the cause.

I sought help from both a dermatologist and an allergist who had me undergo patch testing (all negative) and trials of antihistamines and topical steroids. Without any luck finding a good treatment or diagnosis, I begged my dermatologist for a short-term solution so that I could comfortably visit my daughter while she was studying abroad. Within the first day of beginning my short course of oral prednisone, the itch was gone! I felt so relieved and was able to spend time with my daughter unbothered. However, as soon as I returned and my prednisone ran out, the itch returned in full force. I tried another course of prednisone, but it didn't work as well. More topical steroids? Didn't help either. I desperately needed answers, not more steroids.

After several skin biopsies, I was finally diagnosed with prurigo nodularis and started on a topical preparation of ketamine-amitriptyline-lidocaine (KAL), which was the first nonsteroid treatment that provided me with any relief. However, every night the itch returned—I scratched myself until blood was drawn and ruined many items of clothing and bedding. I even frequently slept on the couch to avoid waking my wife by itching and pacing throughout the night. I returned to the dermatologist in search of a more complete, systemic treatment and tried several that provided me with varied levels of relief: mirtazapine (some), doxepin (none), gabapentin (good relief but felt drowsy), coal tar shampoo (none), and, finally, methotrexate (the most!).

Despite each moment of relief, I was constantly fearful and paranoid that the itch would return. I refused to leave my home for more than a few hours without taking my medications with me and found myself cancelling social plans with others. When I did leave the home, I made sure to wear an undershirt so that if I did scratch myself and draw blood, it would protect my clothing and others from seeing. I started to wash my new clothes several times before ever wearing them because I felt that something about new clothing made it itchier. I saw a holistic/integrated health physician who recommended I test the water and materials in my home, which made me paranoid despite finding nothing during inspections. People would notice me scratching in public and try to offer suggestions for how to handle it, but I didn't want to hear it. I had tried everything.

I was tired, and in search of support from those experiencing similar problems, I joined many prurigo nodularis groups on Facebook. It was there where I first read about dupilumab (Dupixent) and how PN is sometimes related to atopic dermatitis. When I returned to the dermatologist, I asked about this possibility and my dermatologist agreed. We did another biopsy and found histological evidence of underlying atopic dermatitis, and I started on Dupixent the following week. Within one week I noticed my itching had significantly decreased, and within six weeks I was shocked at how little my itch bothered me throughout the day. Now, still on dupilumab, 95% of my itching is eliminated and it only seems to return a few days before my next dose is due. Since starting dupilumab, I am confident leaving my home, socializing, and not planning my life around my itch for the first time in four years. I comfortably sleep through the night next to my wife, wear shirts without undershirts, and can even have a beer or cocktail without worrying too much about my liver like I did when on methotrexate. I admittedly still worry if one day the dupilumab will become less effective, but my quality of life has improved so significantly in the meantime that I am grateful for the present.

My advice to anyone experiencing these same problems, either with prurigo nodularis or a different itchy disease, is that while sometimes it may seem like you are alone, you NEVER are. Any doctor who doesn't believe your itching is real or tells you to "just stop scratching" is not going to help you—continue pursuing other physicians until you find ones that see you, hear you, and will work tirelessly to get you the answers and help you need. I promise, they're out there. While you are going through the tiresome process of searching for a diagnosis or trial-and-erroring different treatments, utilize the support resources that are out there! Join Facebook groups to learn from others' experiences, reach out to family and friends and let them know what is going on, and search for national organizations that advocate for people like you. And finally, whenever you feel too exhausted or fearful to continue, don't give up.

Chronic Spontaneous Urticaria (Hives)

In our "Acute Itch" section, we talked about urticaria (hives) and why they form. While hives can form as a direct reaction to an allergen, such as a food or an environmental trigger, they can also form spontaneously without an identifiable cause or trigger (**idiopathic**). In addition, they may persist for greater than six weeks, occurring on more days than not. This occurs in 0.5–1% of the world's population and is referred to as chronic urticaria (CU). A key diagnostic feature of CU is **symptomatic dermatographism** ("skin writing"), which refers to the immediate formation of an itchy, linear hive following the path of pressure from a blunt object (such as a pen or finger pad) across the skin. Unlike the other itchy skin conditions that involve the immune system, chronic urticaria induces pruritus through the **histaminergic** pathway (discussed in chapter 1.3) and is responsive to antihistaminergic therapies in 40% of the cases. While two of three cases of chronic urticaria are idiopathic and spontaneous, some may be part of a subgroup called *chronic inducible uticaria* that includes different triggers including cholinergic uticaria, which often occurs as a result of body heat and sweating, whether due to exercise,

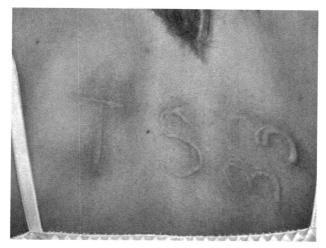

Figure 2.11   Symptomatic dermatographism or "skin writing" in chronic urticaria. Image appears with permission from VisualDx © Logical Images, Inc.

stress, heat from the sun, or certain spicy foods. In this case, the lesions are smaller hive-like lesions that are surrounded by areas of inflamed skin. Additionally, in a smaller number of cases, chronic urticaria may also be associated with autoimmune thyroid disease or the addition of a new medication, supplement, or illicit drug (e.g., opioids).

Lichen Planus

Lichen planus is a common inflammatory disease that causes an itchy rash of the skin or tender lesions in the mouth. Skin lesions of lichen planus are typically pink or purple in color and are typically located on the wrists and ankles. In both the skin and the mouth, lesions of lichen planus often have a lace-like pattern composed of whitish lines known as *Wickham striae*. The cause of lichen planus

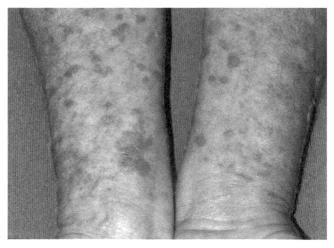

Figure 2.12 Classic presentation of lichen planus with pink/purple papules on the wrists. Image appears with permission from VisualDx © Logical Images, Inc.

is often unknown, but it has been linked to hepatitis C infection in some patients.

Intense itch tends to affect most patients with lichen planus. The itchiest form of lichen planus is known as *hypertrophic lichen planus*, which most often occurs on the lower extremities (usually the shins) and presents as thick **plaques**. Treating both the lesions and itch may involve a variety of therapies, including high-potency topical corticosteroids, tacrolimus, cyclosporine, topical retinoids, and UVB therapy. You can read more about these therapies in chapter 3 of this book.

Pityriasis Rosea
Pityriasis rosea is a **self-limiting** skin rash that often begins with a suddenly appearing, single large lesion known as a *herald patch*. This initial herald patch is often

misdiagnosed as eczema or psoriasis. However, the lesion is often followed one to two weeks later by a more widespread rash lasting for approximately six to eight weeks. This widespread rash is often said to take the distribution of a "Christmas tree." Itch is a frequent complaint in a significant portion of patients with pityriasis rosea and can be severe in a subset of them.

While the herald patch may appear suddenly, it is often preceded by symptoms consistent with a viral upper respiratory infection. This link is often only made in hindsight. While the precise cause of pityriasis rosea is still unclear, this preceding infection suggests that it may be the result of an infectious process. It has previously been linked to human herpesvirus 7 (HHV-7); however, the extent of this association is yet to be determined.

Pityriasis Lichenoides

The rash of pityriasis lichenoides is diffuse and looks similar to psoriasis. It tends to affect mostly adolescents and young adults. While the cause of this rash is still unclear, it has been associated with infections and autoimmunity. It has two forms: the more clinically severe form known as pityriasis lichenoides et varioliformis acuta (PLEVA) and the chronic and more mild form known as pityriasis lichenoides chronica (PLC). PLEVA is characterized by the sudden development of small, scaling **papules** that quickly blister and crust over within a few months. PLC, in contrast, is characterized by a slower, more gradual development of small, scaling papules that may last for a more extended time. Patients with PLEVA often experience intense itch (along with pain and tenderness), while itch is much less common in PLC.

Cutaneous T-Cell Lymphoma

Cutaneous T-cell lymphoma (CTCL) is a rare form of skin cancer that affects the immune system. In the United States, its prevalence is between 16,000 and 20,000 cases. It more commonly occurs in people older than 50 and affects nearly twice as many men as women. Cancer in CTCL originates from cells known as *T lymphocytes*, which are a type of white blood cell that functions to identify and attack infections. In people with CTCL, these T lymphocytes have mutations that cause them to accumulate in the skin. CTCL first appears as lesions in areas of the skin that are usually protected from sun exposure. In lighter-skinned people, these lesions are red and scaly patches. In people with darker skin color, lesions in the skin often appear as either very dark (*hyperpigmented*) or light (*hypopigmented*).

There are several forms of CTCL. Of these, the two most common subtypes of CTCL are **mycosis fungoides** (**MF**) and **Sézary's syndrome**. Studies have revealed that advanced tumoral stages of the cancer and Sézary's syndrome are significantly itchier than patches of skin affected with mycosis fungoides. MF is the most common form of CTCL. People with mycosis fungoides often have localized areas of red, itchy patches in areas protected from the sun that are often confused with eczema or psoriasis. Sézary's syndrome is a more advanced form of MF that is characterized by the spread of mutated T cells into the bloodstream. People with Sézary's syndrome usually have an extremely itchy, scaling red rash that covers most of their body.

Itch in CTCL Itch in CTCL is particularly difficult to treat and intractable. It is often the first and most bother-

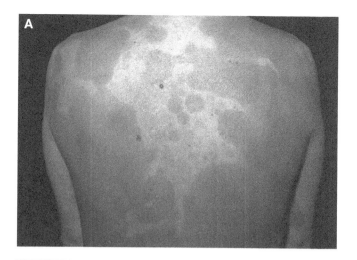

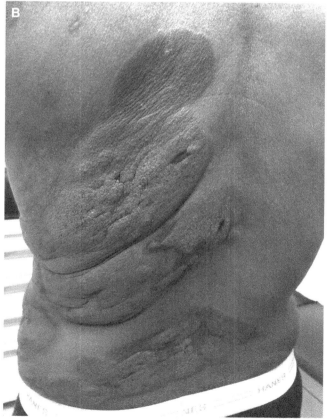

Figure 2.13 (A, B) Two patients with extensive cutaneous T-cell lymphoma (CTCL). Image A appears with permission from VisualDx © Logical Images, Inc. Image B is from the collection of the authors.

some symptom of CTCL, and it can significantly affect quality of life and sleep. Studies have estimated that the incidence of itch in patients with CTCL ranges between 66% and 88%. Itch is more common in people with Sézary's syndrome than in those with mycosis fungoides. It is also significantly more common in later stages of the disease. The itch is usually generalized, but it can also be localized to specific skin lesions. It is thought to be caused by the increased release of certain cytokines by the mutated T lymphocytes.

In general, the management of CTCL-related itch is based on treating the lymphoma. The treatment of the lymphoma is dependent on the stage at which it is diagnosed and may include both topical and systemic therapies.

2.2.3 Itch Associated with Autoimmune Disorders

An autoimmune disorder is any disease where your immune system mistakenly recognizes a part of your body, such as a specific protein, as foreign and forms antibodies against it. These antibodies signal the rest of your immune system to react and attack the healthy target. Depending on whether the targeted protein is located within a specific organ, such as the skin, or throughout the body, the resulting symptoms can be localized or widespread. Below we discuss some of the main autoimmune diseases that impact the skin and cause itch.

Bullous Skin Disorders

Bullous skin disorders refer to the development of blisters, which are collections of fluid between different layers in the skin. These blisters form because the immune system attacks proteins that hold the layers of skin together—when these proteins are attacked, the layers of skin separate. What distinguishes each of these disorders from the others is the layer of skin where the blister forms. The deeper the layer of the skin where the blister forms, the more tense and firm the blister will be. For example, bullous pemphigoid impacts the junction between the epidermis and the dermis, leading to more firm blisters, whereas pemphigus impacts the junction between cells within the epidermis only and leads to softer blisters more prone to rupturing. The different diseases can be grouped based on the level of the skin where blisters form, along with their distribution in the body.

The bullous disorders that are most commonly associated with itch include the following:

- **Bullous pemphigoid (BP).** Blisters in bullous pemphigoid are tense and difficult to break. Bullous pemphigoid often begins with terrible itch that can be generalized or limited to several parts of the body. Itch can precede lesions in BP and is often the most troubling symptom for people who have BP.
- **Dermatitis herpetiformis.** Dermatitis herpetiformis is often associated with gluten intolerance. It is symmetrical and often consists of blisters, **erosions**, and **papules** found commonly on the buttocks, elbows, and knees. Dermatitis herpetiformis is characterized by an extremely severe form of itching. Usually it's not blisters that you see but rather small erosions and **excoriations** that can be confused with eczema or other secondary skin changes. Itch in dermatitis herpetiformis can also appear before the skin lesions.

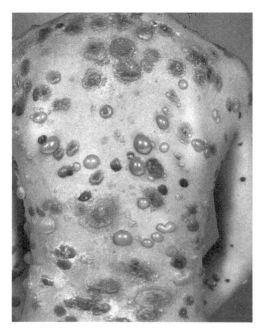

Figure 2.14 Large, fluid-filled blisters in bullous pemphigoid. Image appears with permission from VisualDx © Logical Images, Inc.

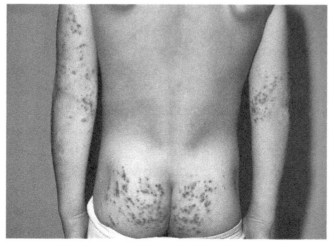

Figure 2.15 Classic lesions of dermatitis herpetiformis featuring intense redness and tiny blisters. Image appears with permission from VisualDx © Logical Images, Inc.

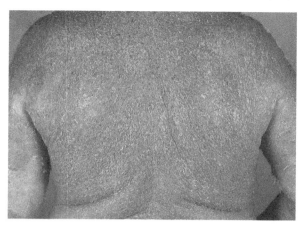

Figure 2.16 Extensive erosions on the back from pemphigus foliaceus. Image appears with permission from VisualDx © Logical Images, Inc.

- **Pemphigus foliaceus.** One of the itchiest autoimmune blistering disorders, pemphigus foliaceus often affects the face and chest and back. Pemphigus foliaceus has blisters that often rupture and leave behind **erosions**.
- **Epidermolysis bullosa congenita.** This is a rare inherited disease (incidence is 1 in 50,000 individuals) that causes the formation of blisters in the skin and mucous membranes. The skin in people with epidermolysis bullosa is extremely fragile, and even minimal trauma or friction can cause significant blistering. There are many genetic variants of epidermolysis bullosa. The dystrophic types are usually extremely itchy. Epidermolysis bullosa pruriginosa is a rare dystrophic variant that produces uncontrollable itching and scratching, often leading to disfiguring skin lesions.

General antipruritic therapies (see chapter 3) are often effective in reducing itch in these disorders. In addition, suppressing the inflammatory response can be a useful tool in treating both the disease and itch.

Dermatomyositis

Dermatomyositis is an inflammatory disease characterized by symmetrical muscle weakness and significant skin rash. The rash in dermatomyositis is aggravated by sun exposure and features a purplish rash usually on the eyelids, face, neck, knuckles, or elbows. Dermatomyositis can be associated with an underlying internal malignancy in some people. Muscle weakness often first affects the hips and shoulders and can cause difficulty in climbing stairs or standing from a sitting position. Itch is one of the most bothersome symptoms encountered by people with dermatomyositis and is often the first symptom of the disease experienced. In general, treatments that reduce inflammation (see chapter 3) are effective for reducing itch along with improving muscle function.

Did You Know?

Gottron's sign, one of the most common skin manifestations of dermatomyositis, manifests as a red, scaly eruption over the knuckles, elbows, or knee joints.

Scleroderma

Scleroderma, also known as systemic sclerosis, is a rare, chronic disease characterized by thickening and scarring

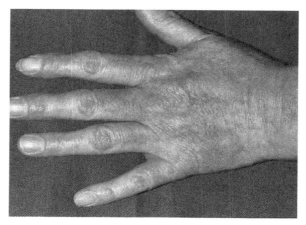

Figure 2.17 Gottron's sign, one of the most common skin manifestations of dermatomyositis, manifests as a red, scaly eruption over the knuckles, elbows, or knee joints. Image appears with permission from VisualDx © Logical Images, Inc.

of the skin. The word "scleroderma" is Greek for "hard skin." This skin thickening can create a loss of flexibility and increase movement difficulties. Additionally, internal organs are often also affected by the underlying disease process. Which organs are affected depends on the scleroderma subtype:

1. Diffuse, which often affects the heart, lungs, and gastrointestinal tract, among other organs; and
2. Limited, which is often referred to as CREST syndrome, and localized to these five key symptoms:
   - Calcinosis: calcium deposits under the skin and sometimes in tissues
   - Raynaud's phenomenon: an exaggerated response to cold temperatures that causes the fingertips and/ or toes to change color (red→ white→ blue), feel numb, or tingle

- Esophageal dysmotility: abnormal movement of the esophagus, often presenting as "heartburn"
- Sclerodactyly: thickened skin on the fingers
- Telangiectasias: enlarged blood vessels that appear as red spots on the fingers, face, or other skin areas

Itch has been reported in 40–50% of patients with scleroderma and can be an extremely bothersome aspect of the disease. Sometimes, this itch is caused by increased skin dryness and can be appropriately treated with topical moisturizers and other emollients. Other times, the itch may be caused by skin inflammation associated with the disease and can be better treated with topical and/or systemic anti-inflammatory agents (see chapter 3).

Sjögren's Syndrome

Sjögren's syndrome is an autoimmune disease in which the body attacks the lubricating glands throughout the body. As such, the skin may become very dry. There is also damage to nerve fibers, which can cause peripheral neuropathy. Treatment includes using over-the-counter emollients and drugs to treat peripheral neuropathies, such as the antiseizure medications gabapentin and pregabalin.

2.2.4 Itch Associated with Infections

Many infections have the potential to cause severe itch. In this chapter, we discuss some of the most common infections that can cause itch.

Scabies

Scabies is an extremely itchy condition that affects as many as 300 million people worldwide. It is characterized by skin infestation of the mite *Sarcoptes scabiei*. This mite is tiny and can burrow and lay its eggs in the skin. Scabies is acquired through direct body-to-body contact with another individual (usually this contact is prolonged). For this reason, it is more common in children attending daycare centers, nursing home residents, and family members of people who are affected with the condition. While the face is spared from scabies, most other areas of the body can be infected. Scabies most commonly affects the skin folds, including the neck, armpits, genitals, and finger web areas.

Scabies can often be difficult for doctors to diagnose, since it often mimics many other skin diseases. If several family members also suffer from severe itch, then a diagnosis of scabies should be made until proven otherwise

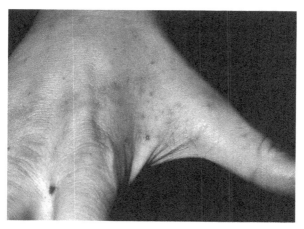

Figure 2.18   Scabies on hands in the folds between the fingers, a common sign that the mites can be found. Image appears with permission from VisualDx © Logical Images, Inc.

(even if the rash does not look classical). When scabies is suspected, doctors often scrape the skin folds of the hands and look under the microscope to see if any mites are present.

Itch in Scabies Severe itching is the hallmark of scabies and is caused by the immune system's response to mite proteins. These proteins can remain in the skin several weeks to months after the mite itself is eliminated with treatment, meaning that the itch of scabies can remain for that long too. This is referred to as *postscabetic itch.* Since the itch in scabies is secondary to an allergic reaction to the protein, if scabies is contracted again, the intense itch will immediately return due to an immune response. In general, itch in scabies tends to be worse later in the day, especially in the evening and at night.

While infected with the mite, treatment aims to eradicate it. This includes medications known as scabicides, such as permethrin cream, oral ivermectin, or crotamiton (known to have a significant effect in reducing itch). Postscabetic itch can be managed with general antipruritic therapies.

Dermatophytosis

Dermatophytes (superficial fungal infections, also known as *tinea infections*, or ringworm) are common causes of itch that is localized to specific body areas. These infections often start as red scaly patches with central clearing or are lighter in color toward the center of the lesion. These infections are especially common in athletes and tend to affect the skin folds, such as in the groin area ("jock itch") and the feet ("athlete's foot"). Factors that increase the risk for developing one of these infections include clothing that is tight-fitting, warm temperatures, and moisture. Itch associated with tinea infections can be severe and cause significant distress.

Did You Know?

Another name for dermatophytosis is ringworm, but this is a misnomer! The infection isn't caused by worms at all but rather is the result of a fungal infection.

Treatment for itch associated with fungal infections is directed against the underlying cause. Common topical antifungals include miconazole, terbinafine, and clotrimazole. In more severe cases (or in infections affecting the scalp or nails), systemic treatment with oral antifungal medications is used.

Folliculitis

Folliculitis is the infection of one or more hair follicles and can occur anywhere on the skin that hair is present. It occurs when hair follicles become infected with *Staph* bacteria (short for *Staphylococcus*), often through touching, rubbing, or shaving. Pimples or pustules (bumps filled with pus) are the result of these infected follicles. Itch in folliculitis is due to inflammation that occurs as a result of the infection. In addition, *Staphylococcus* bacteria can secrete and activate **proteases** that also induce itch (see chapter 1.2). Warm compresses may help drain the infected follicles, but the best treatment for folliculitis is antibacterial therapy. Common topical antibiotics used to treat folliculitis include clindamycin and mupirocin.

Did You Know?

Folliculitis—an infection of hair follicles that is caused by the bacterium *Staphylococcus aureus*—is known as a "hot tub rash" and associated with sitting in dirty hot tubs.

Human Immunodeficiency Virus

Itch is a common complaint of people with human immunodeficiency virus (HIV) (affecting between 30% and 60% of patients) and can be associated with HIV at many points of infection. Most commonly, itch is an

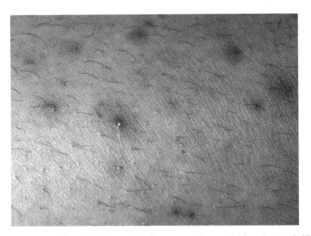

Figure 2.19 Folliculitis, or inflammation of the hair follicle, on the trunk. Image appears with permission from VisualDx © Logical Images, Inc.

initial symptom or it presents as a consequence of dry skin, which is a significant problem in people with HIV.

Primary skin disorders that are particularly common in patients with HIV include psoriasis and seborrheic dermatitis (dandruff). Often, people present with itchy bumps of unknown origin—these can range from hypersensitivity reactions to insect bites to a disease that is particularly associated with advanced HIV known as *eosinophilic folliculitis*. This condition is characterized by small bumps that often affect many areas of the skin, including the trunk, back, face, and extremities. Treatment of the HIV infection with highly active antiretroviral therapy (HAART) usually leads to improvement/resolution of the itch.

Onchocerciasis

Onchocerciasis is an infectious disease caused by the parasite *Onchocerca volvulus* (a roundworm). Most of these infections occur in sub-Saharan Africa (in fact, there are no reported cases in the Western Hemisphere). Around 18 million people suffer from this disease in Africa. This disease is known to cause intense, severe itching, although its most well-known aftereffect is blindness. Oral ivermectin is the treatment of choice and can kill the parasite.

"Traveler's Itch"

Skin diseases may affect up to 8% of people who travel internationally. About 25% of these are infected by what we refer to as "tropical diseases," or diseases more commonly contracted within tropical climates, while the other 74% are bacterial and viral infections that are equally likely to be contracted in nontropical areas. Two of the most common examples of posttravel itching are swimmer's itch and seabather's eruption.

Swimmer's Itch Swimmer's itch, also known as lake itch, often appears as itchy, red bumps on the lower extremities. These skin lesions are the result of an immune reaction by the body against a waterborne parasite known as *Schistosomatidae*. The larvae of these parasites enter the skin. Once in the skin, these larvae immediately die and cause a reaction by the immune system that is often associated with significant inflammation. Each red bump corresponds to an area where a single parasite has invaded the skin.

Seabather's Eruption Seabather's eruption is an extremely itchy rash that occurs underneath the bathing suits of people who swim and dive in the sea in tropical areas. It is

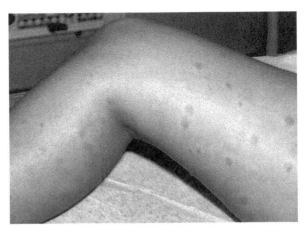

Figure 2.20   Swimmer's itch on the lower extremities. Image appears with permission from VisualDx © Logical Images, Inc.

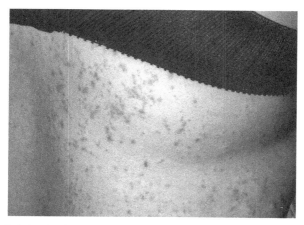

Figure 2.21 Seabather's eruption under the breast. Image appears with permission from VisualDx © Logical Images, Inc.

caused by a hypersensitivity reaction to the larval form of jellyfish.

Additionally, other causes of travel-related itch can be found in table 2.2.

2.2.5 Itch Associated with Systemic Disease

Diseases that affect the internal organs can cause intense, generalized pruritus that typically is not associated with a primary skin rash. Instead, people with itch associated with a systemic disease typically have visible secondary signs of scratching. These may include excoriations, lichenification, or prurigo nodules.

Chronic Kidney Disease–Associated Pruritus
Chronic kidney disease (CKD) can cause associated itch. The term "chronic kidney disease" is sometimes used interchangeably with end-stage renal failure (ESRF), which

Table 2.2 Causes of Travel-Related Itch

Diagnosis	Travel/traveler risk factors	Presentation
Insect bites	Worldwide; lack of repellents, protective clothing, nets	*Localized itch.* Red bumps, blisters, or hives; bites in clusters (often threes) or lines
Cutaneous larva migrans	Tropics, especially Caribbean; beach holidays; walking barefoot or sitting on sandy soil; preponderance in children and teenagers	*Localized itch.* Serpiginous (snake-like), moving tract; most commonly on feet > buttocks > trunk
Allergic reaction	Worldwide; underlying atopic dermatitis, asthma, or other allergies; exposure to medications, foods, animals, plants, arthropods	*Diffuse itch.* Hives, swelling
Fungal skin infection	Worldwide, especially the tropics; exposure to animals, sweat, heat, moisture, communal bathrooms	*Localized itch.* Erythematous plaques or scales, annular lesions, pigment change; body folds
Scabies	Worldwide, especially tropics; poor crowded conditions; backpackers, aid workers; skin-to-skin contact, sexual contact	*Diffuse itch* (worse at night); burrows in web spaces, wrists, elbows, axillae, genitalia; generalized rash
Swimmer's itch (cercarial dermatitis)	Worldwide (Africa, Middle East, Asia, South America for human ones); immersion in fresh water	*Localized itch.* Red papules, sometimes blisters or hives; exposed skin

Table 2.2 (Continued)

Diagnosis	Travel/traveler risk factors	Presentation
Seabather's eruption	Tropical and subtropical coastal destinations, especially US, Caribbean, Latin America, Papua New Guinea, Singapore, and Philippines; swimming and surfing trips; summer	*Localized itch.* Skin rash in areas typically covered by swimming attire
Phytophoto-dermatitis-Berloque dermatitis	Worldwide; beach holidays; skin exposure to UV light and sensitizing botanical agents (lime, other citrus fruits, celery)	*Localized itch* (mild). Painful burning erythema, then blisters, then painless, dark-colored streaky lesions; do not migrate
Ciguatera poisoning	Worldwide, especially Pacific, Caribbean, Indian Ocean; ingestion of fish carrying ciguatoxin (barracuda, mackerel, snapper, tuna)	*Diffuse itch.* Associated gastrointestinal and neurological symptoms (e.g., hot/cold temperature reversal); symptoms worsen following alcohol
Invasive phase of parasitic diseases	Mostly seen in immigrants or long-term travelers to developing and tropical regions	Variable

refers to people with stage 5 CKD who are close to requiring dialysis or are currently undergoing dialysis. However, in recent years, we have come to understand that itch in CKD affects more than just those on dialysis or with ESRF. Rather, it has been shown to occur as early as stage 3 CKD and increases in prevalence with worsening kidney function, age, and medical comorbidities.

Overall, 20–40% of patients with CKD report intense, generalized itching that is moderate to severe. This itch is usually generalized but can be especially severe on the back and the extremities. It can significantly affect quality of life, sleep, and mood. People with ESRF itch often have secondary signs of scratching such as heavily excoriated skin, lichenification, and prurigo nodules.

The cause of CKD pruritus is still incompletely understood but seems to be a combination of imbalances in the immune and opioid systems, damage to nerve fibers transmitting itch, the release of **cytokines** during hemodialysis, and an abnormality in a number of laboratory values such as calcium and phosphorus that may be altered in people with chronic renal disease who are undergoing hemodialysis. Patients who undergo kidney transplantation, and thus no longer require hemodialysis, often no longer experience the intense itch they once lived with. However, for those awaiting transplantation or those who are not a transplant candidate, itch in CKD is treated by targeting these potential underlying causes. The dialysis regimen may be altered by the physician to maximize clearance of toxins and normalize laboratory values. Gabapentin and pregabalin can be used to quiet damaged nerves and decrease the sensation of itch. New, emerging treatments specifically designed for itch in CKD include kappa opioids that seek to restore the body's natural opioid balance (see chapter 3.3.4). In addition, good skin hygiene (see chapter 3.1) is key in patients with itch in CKD, as many of these patients have dry skin that can further increase itch.

Cholestatic Itch (Liver Disease Itch)

Cholestasis occurs when the flow of bile ("chole") from your liver is decreased or blocked ("stasis")—this can occur secondary to any disease affecting the liver. As such, *cholestatic itch* refers to itch associated with chronic liver disease. This itch is unique in that it often starts in the palms and soles and spreads to other body sites. Specific liver diseases associated with itch include hepatitis C, primary biliary cirrhosis (more common in women), intrahepatic cholestasis of pregnancy, and obstruction of the bile duct as a complication of cancers of the pancreas or biliary system.

The exact cause of this itch is currently unknown. However, studies have suggested a role for elevated levels of bile salts and opioid levels. Therefore, appropriate treatments target these factors. Two therapies specific for pruritus of cholestasis include compounds that bind bile acids to lower their levels (examples are cholestyramine and ursodeoxycholic acid). In addition, drugs that block mu-opioid receptors (e.g., naltrexone) and drugs that activate kappa-opioid receptors and restore an opioid balance (e.g., butorphanol) are useful in decreasing itch. Combining these treatments may be particularly helpful. Of course, treating the underlying cause of chronic liver disease or undergoing a liver transplantation would also help relieve cholestatic pruritus.

Pruritus Associated with Endocrine Disorders

Disturbances in the endocrine system have the potential to cause significant itch and distress. Endocrine conditions that have been associated with pruritus are listed below. The best treatment for itch associated with these conditions is better disease control of the underlying condition.

Two conditions that can be associated with itch are thyroid problems and diabetes. While the exact mechanism is unknown, **hyperthyroidism** is more commonly associated with itch than hypothyroidism. **Diabetes** is a disease that results from increased levels of blood sugars. It has many potential complications, such as infections and damage to nerve fibers (neuropathy). One common infection that is known to cause itch in uncontrolled diabetes is **candidal (yeast) infection,** which most commonly occurs in skin folds and the anogenital region. It appears as a rapidly expanding red rash.

Neuropathy is a common complication in people with diabetes that can cause significant itch. One presentation for itch associated with diabetic neuropathy is localized itch that tends to affect the scalp and lower extremities. A large study from Japan showed that people with diabetic neuropathy have an increased frequency of itch affecting the trunk. Drugs that target the nerves and neuropathy such as topical local anesthetics (e.g., lidocaine), capsaicin, and oral antiseizure treatments like gabapentin and pregabalin are often helpful.

Pruritus Associated with Blood Disorders

Itch is a very common symptom in people with blood disorders. One form of blood disorder, cutaneous T-cell lymphoma, was discussed earlier. Other lymphomas associated with itch include **Hodgkin's** and **non-Hodgkin's lymphoma**. Itch has also been associated with leukemias and other forms of erratic red and white blood cell production known as *myelodysplasia*.

Did You Know?

Sometimes chronic itch can be a symptom of cancer, more commonly in lymphomas and blood disorders. This condition has been called paraneoplastic pruritus.

Polycythemia vera is another blood disorder that is highly associated with itch, occurring in approximately half of all people with the condition. Itch in polycythemia vera is unique in that it is made worse and often triggered by exposure to water (*aquagenic pruritus*). The cause of itch in polycythemia vera is unknown; it has been associated with increased levels of histamine.

Drug-Associated Pruritus

Numerous pharmacologic drugs can induce generalized pruritus in patients through a variety of mechanisms, including drug rashes, dry skin, alteration of neural pathways, phototoxicity, cholestatic liver injury, and dilation of blood vessels. A temporal (time-based) relationship between the addition of any new drugs and the onset of itch is the clearest way to determine the offending agent.

In addition, the abuse of several substances, such as stimulants (e.g., cocaine, amphetamines, attention-deficit/hyperactivity disorder medications, etc.) and mu opioids (prescribed or nonprescribed), can result in itch. Opioid-induced pruritus typically presents as a generalized pruritus. On the other hand, central nervous system stimulant misuse may present with a feeling of bugs or parasites crawling underneath the skin. Itch can present as a result of use of these substances even when the drug is prescribed and being used correctly.

2.2.6 Neuropathic Itch

Neuropathic itch, or nerve itch, includes a broad group of conditions in which itch is caused by damage to nerve fibers. Any localized itch with limited body involvement and without rash should raise the suspicion of neuropathic itch. This damage can occur at different levels and can be classified into two categories: peripheral and central. Peripheral nerve fiber damage can be defined as damage to nerves occurring at any point beyond the spinal cord where the nerves branch out, whereas central nerve fiber damage includes any damage to nerves in the spinal cord or brain.

Peripheral Neuropathic Itch

Postherpetic Neuralgia Postherpetic neuralgia classically features pain in certain parts of the body as a result of nerve damage caused by the varicella zoster virus—the virus that causes chickenpox in children and shingles in adults. This virus can lie dormant in a person's nervous system for many years and can reactivate in approximately 10–20% of adults, causing severe burning pain and neuropathic itch. Itch is more common in the face, neck, and head. The best treatments for itch associated with postherpetic neuralgia are medications specifically targeting the nerves, like gabapentin and pregabalin, and topical anesthetics, like lidocaine and capsaicin.

Brachioradial Pruritus Brachioradial pruritus is a localized itch of the upper arms, forearms, and elbows that can start in one or both arms. It seems to originate as a spinal nerve pathology affecting the cervical (neck) nerve roots (those thought to be responsible for symptoms are located between the C4 and C7 cervical vertebrae). It specifically worsens in the summer months, which is thought to be caused by increased exposure to sunlight. In addition, many patients find relief of their itch when an ice pack or cooling agent is applied to the affected area. Sometimes, this itch can spread to the rest of the body. Topical treatments that may be especially effective for patients with brachioradial pruritus include local anesthetics (such as lidocaine, prilocaine, or pramoxine) and topical capsaicin and topical ketamine-lidocaine-amitriptyline. Systemic treatments, such as gabapentin and pregabalin, are often successfully used (see chapter 3.3.2).

Notalgia Paresthetica Notalgia paresthetica is a form of chronic itch that is localized to the infrascapular area on the back, that is, the triangular area between your scapula and your spine. People with notalgia paresthetica have an intense urge to scratch the area underneath the shoulder blade. In addition to itch, people can experience tingling and burning sensations, and the area is sometimes hyperpigmented (dark) as a consequence of chronic scratching.

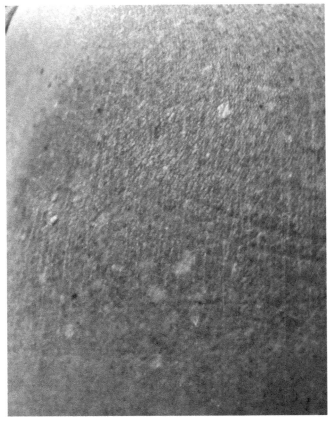

Figure 2.22 Hyperpigmented patch on the back in notalgia paresthetica. Author photo.

Similar to brachioradial pruritus, notalgia paresthetica originates with pressure on spinal nerves (ranging from degenerative changes in the spine to nerve impingement). Here the thoracic nerves are affected (the specific nerves affected are thought to be located between thoracic vertebrae T2 and T6). Topical treatments usually provide some relief in people with notalgia paresthetica and include capsaicin and local anesthetics like pramoxine.

In severe itch, oral gabapentin and pregabalin can be effective treatments. Physical therapy may also provide some relief.

My Experience with Brachioradial Pruritus

By Denis Eirikis

I handle pain well. As a US Coast Guard lieutenant, I served steadfastly in harm's way as a first responder to everything from ship fires to chemical spills. I have taken hard punches in the face as an amateur boxer. I've undergone painful bone fusion surgery. I once even walked away from a US Marines helicopter crash and went on with my mission, but I have never in my life ever experienced anything as miserable and terrifying as brachioradial pruritus (BRP).

Imagine an electrical sensation starting deep within your arms. It's part itch, part pain; it's a combination of pins and needles, burning and tingling. It's unlike anything else you've felt before. You can't relieve it by scratching, but in your sleep you try anyway. You twitch, feel electrical zaps, try scratching again (violently this time). In half sleep, you now feel the sensations of a phantom army of stinging red ants impossibly burrowed into your arm. You scream yourself awake, but the horror doesn't stop. Your arms are scratched bloody. Your sleep-deprived mate is looking at you like you are crazy. Worst of all, that horrifying deep itch is still there.

This is what I and many others suffering from BRP have experienced.

My first experience with BRP occurred around 2016 at the age of 63. After a full summer of hiking every other day in the midday South Florida sun, I started to feel a "deep itch" within both of my arms. Knowing nothing else, I began to think my deeply tanned, olive-skinned arms were no longer immune from the sun's rays and started using sunblock for the first time. The sensation faded, and I thought I had solved my minor problem—I was wrong.

In September 2020, I had one of the worst experiences with my own body. After another summer of biking, hiking, and spending countless hours in the midday South Florida sun, I began to feel a deep undulating itch in both of my arms. For several weeks I couldn't sleep, scratched myself bloody throughout the night, and fantasized about taking knives to my own skin to relieve myself of this pain below its surface. My mental health deteriorated, and I catastrophized that this pain would last the rest of my life.

After this flare, I've had numerous others ranging in severity from mild to intolerable. However, I am thrilled to say that I have not had a flare for over a year. Through many series of trails and errors of treatments ranging from pharmacologic to psychologic, I've found what works best for me. But, as webmaster for BRPalliance.org, it is very apparent that managing BRP is not a "one-size-fits-all" approach. BRP is not only a product of nerve damage somewhere along the spine-to-arms pathway (known as the brachioradial nerve), but also how our brains interpret the signals from these damaged nerves. Some people find that treatments designed to quiet these nerve signals (topical ketamine/amitriptyline/lidocaine, oral gabapentin, etc.) are very effective. I personally did not—rather, I found that focusing on the way I perceived my itch was most beneficial.

I began to think of BRP as "itch hallucination." At the first sensations of BRP itch, I remember that it is just my brain's interpretation of nerve signals. I use **mindfulness** to explore the itch, remind myself that perception is something I can control, and then intentionally dismiss the itch and use mindfulness to think of something else. I have also found icing my arms to be incredibly beneficial—perhaps by numbing some of the sensation coming from them, but also maybe causing a distraction from the itch my brain is perceiving.

In any case, identifying BRP triggers and avoiding them is a key part of BRP management. However, like in other aspects of BRP management, this is also not "one size fits all." For me, I've noticed that my main trigger is sunlight, and through covering up my arms when biking, not just with SPF but also with long-sleeved clothing, I have seen significant improvements. For others, vibration is a major trigger and can be useful to avoid.

My big takeaway from my own experience with BRP and interacting with the larger BRP patient community is that different things work for different people. I encourage patients new to BRP to gravitate toward solutions they believe will work for them because if you think it will work, there's a much better chance that it will. While the trial and error of different management plans may be time-consuming and stressful, it is important to not lose hope. In my darkest times and most severe flares, I never dreamt that my current flare-free state would be achievable. It will get better.

Central Neuropathic Itch

Central neuropathic itch involves pathology in the brain or spinal cord. Descriptions of two examples of central causes of itch follow.

Multiple Sclerosis Multiple sclerosis is an autoimmune disease in which the fatty sheath around nerve fibers in the spinal cord and brain is damaged. We recently found that 40% of people with multiple sclerosis experience spontaneous outbreaks of itch that can occur for seconds to minutes. This itch may be either localized or generalized usually in the upper and lower extremities.

Stroke Numerous brain areas have been found to be associated with itch. Thus, a lack of oxygen delivery to brain tissue in the areas involved in itch sensation can lead to significant neuropathic itch.

Phantom Itch

Phantom itch is a sensation that can occur after the amputation of a limb or other body part, such that the patient continues to feel sensations in that missing part. It is rare that phantom itch is experienced in the absence of phantom pain. Many of the same therapies used to treat phantom pain have been shown effective in treating phantom itch. Prosthetics that provide visual and functional stimulation, mechanical stimulation, and "mirror therapy" (using the opposite limb and a mirror to simulate movement of the missing limb) have all been shown to be effective. In addition, treatment with systemic therapies like gabapentin, pregabalin, and tricyclic antidepressants may also be useful.

2.2.7 Pruritus in the Elderly

The incidence of chronic itch tends to increase as patients get older. In fact, it has been estimated that 25% of geriatric outpatients and nursing home residents experience chronic itch. Itch in patients over the age of 65 can have a variety of causes. Generalized dry skin is extremely common due to a decrease in skin thickness and moisture as we age. Common conditions such as seborrheic dermatitis, contact dermatitis, nummular eczema, and psoriasis are also common in the elderly. In addition, the increasing number of systemic diseases and disorders such as chronic

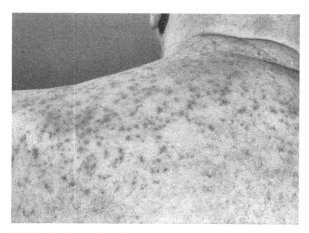

Figure 2.23   Itchy red rash in Grover's disease. Image appears with permission from VisualDx © Logical Images, Inc.

kidney disease and liver disease as we age may also contribute to chronic itch in the elderly (see chapter 2.2.5).

Grover's disease, or transient acantholytic dermatosis, is a very itchy rash made up of papules and vesicles located mainly on the trunk and extremities. It most commonly affects elderly Caucasian men and can be exacerbated by sunlight, hot temperatures, and sweat. While this condition is usually benign in nature, it has sometimes been associated with malignancies and reactions to skin infections.

In some cases of chronic itch in patients over the age of 65, there is not an identifiable inflammatory, systemic, or neuropathic cause. This is referred to as **chronic pruritus of aging** and is considered its own entity. In this condition, primary skin findings like rash are uncommon, and if skin findings do exist, they are frequently secondary skin changes like excoriations from scratching. While the exact cause of this condition is unknown, several physiological changes that occur in the skin as we age may contribute. These changes include a decrease in skin thickness and moisture, a gradual worsening of immune system function (known as *immunosenescence*, or aging of the immune system, which can result in greater amounts of inflammation), and the frequent copresence of psychological and neurodegenerative disorders. In addition, age-related changes in nerve fibers and feelings of social isolation may exacerbate itch in this population.

2.2.8 Chronic Pruritus of Unknown Origin

Chronic pruritus of unknown origin (CPUO), sometimes also referred to as idiopathic pruritus or generalized pruritus of undetermined origin (GPUO), is the term used to describe a disorder of chronic itching for which an extensive workup for other causes has been completed and still no clear underlying cause is uncovered. Before this diagnosis is made, a careful evaluation should be made by your doctor to exclude both dermatologic and nondermatologic causes of your pruritus. These include the following:

- Physical examination should evaluate for the presence of primary skin lesions (for example, lesions associated with atopic dermatitis, psoriasis, or cutaneous T-cell lymphoma).
- Systemic causes for pruritus should be excluded by performing the following laboratory tests:
  ◦ *Complete blood count (CBC).* This test looks at the different types of blood cells in the body (including red and white blood cells as well as platelets). An abnormality in these tests can alert the physician to hematologic abnormalities or clues about other types of underlying systemic disease.
  ◦ *Liver function tests (LFTs).* It is important to make sure that there are no abnormalities in the liver and the associated biliary system, since they can be a cause of itch.
  ◦ *Blood urea nitrogen/creatinine.* Any of these studies (if abnormal) can alert the physician to pathologies related to the kidney.
  ◦ *Thyroid function tests.* These studies can alert the physician to the presence of abnormal functioning of the thyroid gland. Hyperthyroidism is more commonly associated with chronic itch than is hypothyroidism.

- *Chest x-ray.* A chest x-ray may alert the physicians to underlying malignancies responsible for the chronic itch.

The following tests may also be indicated, based on your physician's concerns and your medical history:

- HIV serology
- Stool studies for ova and parasites
- Iron studies (to look for iron-deficiency anemia, as it has been associated with chronic itch)
- Computed tomography (CT) scan of the chest or abdomen when a lymphoma or other malignancy is suspected
- Magnetic resonance imaging (MRI) of the spine in people who are suspected to have a neuropathic itch, particularly brachioradial pruritus and notalgia paresthetica

Despite the inability to identify an underlying cause in CPUO, it does not mean that treatment of itch is impossible. In fact, many general systemic antipruritic treatments have been shown to be effective in treating CPUO. These treatments are discussed in further detail in chapter 3 of this book.

2.2.9 Pruritus in Pregnancy and Menopause

Pregnancy

Many people experience a significant increase in itch during pregnancy, but the underlying mechanism is unknown. Recent studies in rats suggest that the female sex hormones estrogen and estradiol have a significant role in inducing itch in pregnancy.

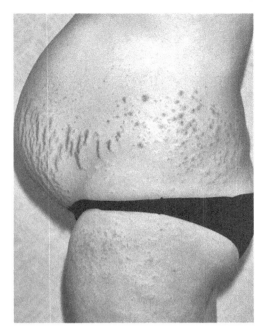

Figure 2.24 Polymorphic eruption of pregnancy is an itchy rash that develops during the third trimester of pregnancy. It commonly begins on the abdomen, particularly within stretch marks. Image appears with permission from VisualDx © Logical Images, Inc.

Several specific itchy conditions can develop throughout pregnancy. Below we discuss some of the more common ones:

• **Polymorphic eruption of pregnancy,** also known as pruritic urticarial papules and plaques of pregnancy, is characterized by very itchy welts and hives of the skin that typically begin in stretch marks located on the abdomen. It is associated with multiparous pregnancies (i.e., twins, triplets, etc.). This rash typically occurs in late pregnancy or postpartum and usually resolves by six weeks after delivery.

- **Pemphigoid gestationis** is a rare autoimmune disease that involves the formation of very itchy red blisters and hives. In many cases, the itch may begin before the appearance of skin lesions. This condition usually occurs in the third trimester or immediately postpartum and has a tendency to flare at the time of delivery. The condition typically resolves within weeks of delivery.

- **Intrahepatic cholestasis of pregnancy** is a condition that frequently occurs late in pregnancy and is not associated with primary skin lesions. Instead, it is the result of an inability to effectively secrete bile salts (and is often diagnosed by an elevation of bile acids in the blood). Itch often occurs suddenly and starts on the palms of the hands or soles of the feet before quickly generalizing to the rest of the body. A specific treatment is ursodeoxycholic acid, which reduces serum bile acid levels.

- **Atopic eruption of pregnancy** is a condition that is associated with eczematous changes in the skin, although preexisting atopic dermatitis is not a requirement. Unlike the other conditions mentioned above, atopic eruptions in pregnancy tend to occur earlier in the course of a pregnancy. Lesions take many forms and are often extremely itchy. Women with this condition often respond well to topical corticosteroids.

Menopause

Menopause is associated with a decrease in the amount of estrogen in the skin and with changes in vaginal acidity (pH).

Atrophic vulvovaginitis is an itchy condition that can occur in menopausal and postmenopausal women and is associated with thinning of the vagina due to a decrease in estrogen levels. Many women with this condition quickly respond to topical therapy with estrogen.

Lichen sclerosus is another condition that occurs more commonly after menopause and can affect the mucus membranes and skin. It may appear as whitening and thinning of the skin and white scar-like lesions around the openings of the vagina and anus. Lichen sclerosus can be very itchy and is treated with topical corticosteroids (often the more potent types).

2.2.10 Other Causes of Itch

Itch and Burns or Scars

Scars from burns are highly associated with itch. Estimates of prevalence rates of itch three months after a burn injury are as high as 80–90%. The more extensive the burn, the longer the postburn itch might last. Both topical and oral therapies can be considered for treatment of this condition, and research to determine the best treatment methods is ongoing. Laser treatment also can be a therapeutic option for those experiencing itch secondary to burns.

Itch and Keloids

Keloids are a type of scar that results in an overgrowth of scar tissue at the site of a healed skin injury. Keloids often expand beyond the borders of a typical scar into normal skin and can be associated with a significant amount of itch, which is most common at the peripheral

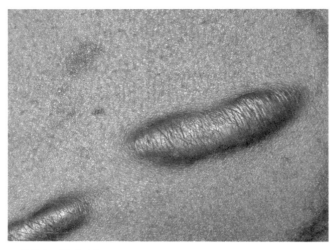

Figure 2.25 Keloid scars. Image appears with permission from VisualDx © Logical Images, Inc.

border of lesions. Research is still ongoing to understand the most effective ways to treat this condition, but current options include intralesional (injected) corticosteroids, occlusion with silicone gel sheets, topical chemotherapy with 5-fluorouracil, cryotherapy, and even laser therapy.

Acne

Acne is a common condition that can affect people throughout the life span but is most common during adolescence. The itch is usually of mild to moderate severity. Indeed, a large Norwegian population study showed a significant correlation between the severity of acne and the intensity of itch. An explanation for this association is that severe acne is often inflammatory. In addition, the organism that causes acne is *Cutibacterium acnes*, which also produces many **proteases** that can activate the **PAR-2 receptor** (a known cause of itch, discussed in chapter 1.3).

Treating the underlying acne using topical and/or oral treatments (antibiotics, vitamin A analogues, etc.) will be most effective for this condition.

Itch and Skin Cancer

Itch is a common feature accompanying nonmelanoma skin cancer, which includes both **basal cell** and **squamous cell carcinoma**.

2.2.11 Itch beyond the Skin

While it may not be a familiar sensation to you, it is possible to experience itch in other organs besides the skin. That's right—other organs such as the eyes, ears, and nose can all experience itch! While some skin conditions (atopic dermatitis, seborrheic dermatitis, and psoriasis) may simply extend into these regions, other conditions that can cause itch are unique to these regions. For example, allergic conditions like **allergic rhinitis** (inflammation of the nose mucosa; also known as seasonal allergies or hay fever) and **conjunctivitis** (inflammation of the eye conjunctiva) can produce itch in the nose and eyes through similar mechanisms as other conditions on the skin (damage to the epithelium, activation of the immune system, and neural damage/sensitization). Below we will discuss some of the more common conditions that can cause itch in each of these organs:

- Eyes
  - *Dry eye syndrome (keratoconjunctivitis sicca).* This is a disorder of the tear film that occurs either due to a deficiency of tears or excessive tear evaporation. One

in seven individuals over the age of 65 years experiences dry eye at some point. This condition can be caused by a variety of etiologies, including neuropathic damage and nerve sensitization, environmental conditions (cigarette smoke exposure), hormonal imbalances, eyelid inflammation, contact lens wear, and systemic disorders (systemic lupus erythematosus [SLE] and Sjögren's syndrome). Management of this condition involves treating the underlying causes, but artificial tears can help manage itchy symptoms in all cases.

○ *Allergic conjunctivitis.* Approximately 40% of the general population is affected by allergic eye disease. While most patients experience bilateral conjunctival injection (redness), ocular itch is the main symptom of this condition and also considered the most debilitating by patients. While rubbing the eyes often provides patients with immediate, short-term relief, it can actually increase the duration and intensity of itching. The best treatment for this condition is eye drops that include both an antihistamine and a mast cell stabilizer, such as olopatadine. Cold compresses and/or lubricant eye drops may also be helpful.

○ *Ocular rosacea.* Rosacea is a condition typically characterized by facial flushing, dilation of capillaries in skin, and inflammatory papules that typically occurs on the face, but ocular lesions can occur in anywhere from 3–58% of patients. Patients often experience both redness and burning of the eyes, as well as itching and dryness. This condition can be treated with oral doxycycline or minocycline, which are inhibitors of the PAR2 receptor that is implicated in chronic itch.

- Ears
  - *Itchy ear syndrome.* This condition consists of itching, burning, prickling, and pain of the external auditory canal (the part you see) without any clinical findings on exam. The underlying mechanism of this condition remains unclear. Treatment generally includes short-term symptomatic control with topical steroids to decrease pruritus.
- Nose
  - *Allergic rhinitis (seasonal allergies/hay fever).* This condition is extremely prevalent, affecting 20–40 million people in the US alone. Nasal itching is a characteristic symptom of this condition in addition to sneezing, congestion, and rhinorrhea (runny nose), so much so that the "allergic salute," or the repetitive action of wiping the nose upward with the wrist or palm, often leads to the "allergic crease," a horizontal crease on the nasal bridge, a key physical finding in these patients. Itching is thought to be due to activation of the **trigeminal nerve** within the nasal mucosa. This condition is often associated with both asthma and atopic dermatitis as part of the **allergic triad** (see chapter 2.2.2). Nasal or oral antihistamines are a mainstay of treatment for this condition.
- Mouth
  - *Oral allergy syndrome (OAS).* OAS, the most common cause of mouth itching, can also include itching of the throat and tongue after consuming certain

foods. This is secondary to cross-reactivity between proteins in some fresh fruits, vegetables, and nuts with pollens. This occurs in up to 70% of people with a pollen allergy. These specific proteins that cross-react with pollens can be broken down with cooking or processing. Therefore, OAS does not typically occur when eating baked fruits/vegetables or processed foods such as applesauce. Symptoms are typically mild, usually only lasting for a few seconds to a few minutes, and rarely progress to a more serious allergic reaction. However, studies have shown that up to 2% of people who experience OAS may develop anaphylaxis a life threatening allergic reaction that can affect all the body. Therefore, it is recommended to undergo an evaluation with an allergist if you experience such symptoms and be cautious if continuing to eat triggering foods.

2.2.12 Itch and the Brain

Itch is highly associated with the brain and mental processes. Researchers have found that simply thinking about itch or watching another person itching will cause you to scratch. Emotional stress can also induce or aggravate itch. Indeed, there is an interrelationship between itch and chronic stress, sleep deprivation, and anxiety/depression—all of which may exacerbate itch of a known etiology or may cause itch independently.

A study found that patients with atopic dermatitis experienced more intense itch than usual while they watched videos of others scratching. An explanation for this finding could be that watching others scratching could cause people distress by bringing back memories of severe scratching episodes. The act of scratching has in turn been suggested as a way for people to provide temporary relief for their inner tensions. These examples illustrate the enhanced role psychological factors play in the perception of itch among people with especially itchy conditions such as atopic dermatitis and psoriasis. In addition, studies have shown that people with chronic itch have a significantly greater level of anxiety and depression. In extreme cases, severe itch could lead to suicidal thoughts.

In particular, depression has been found to correlate with the intensity of itch in people suffering from atopic dermatitis, chronic urticaria, and psoriasis. Studies have also shown that people with depression can suffer severe itch that often responds to common antidepressant medications including tricyclic antidepressants (TCAs), noradrenergic selective serotoninergic antidepressants (NaSSAs), and selective serotonin reuptake inhibitors (SSRIs). Mirtazapine, an NaSSA, may be particularly effective, as it has been shown to significantly reduce itch (especially nighttime itch) and to decrease both anxiety and depressive symptoms. Like people who have depression, people who have fibromyalgia (a common syndrome with depressive symptoms, widespread pain, and lack of sleep) may also have chronic itch.

When talking about psychosocial issues, it is important to also mention how poor social support affects skin diseases. Studies have shown a clear inverse relationship between the amount of social support people have and the intensity of itch that they experience; in other words, people who have better social support experience less severe itch. An explanation for this finding may simply be that increased social support can significantly reduce the amount of stress people experience in their life.

Do You Want to Learn More?

See online supplement for an interactive graphic on how itch can come from damage along any point of the nervous system and brain.

Psychogenic Itch

Psychogenic pruritus is diagnosed by clinicians when no skin pathology or underlying medical disease can be identified but when severe itch is experienced. People with psychogenic pruritus may have associated psychiatric disorders or may recently have experienced significant events in their lives causing psychological distress. Psychogenic pruritus without any other identifiable etiology has an incidence of about 2%. These people have significant amounts of skin excoriation and thickening of the skin known as *lichenification*. While the exact mechanism behind itch of psychogenic origin is unknown, it is likely that an alteration in chemicals in the brain, such as neurotransmitters (for example, serotonin, acetylcholine, epinephrine, and dopamine) and naturally occurring opioids, plays a significant role. They may significantly benefit from psychoactive drugs, including antidepressants, as well as from psychotherapy.

One rare cause of psychogenic itch is called *delusion of infestations.* In this disorder, people have a strong belief that they are infected by parasites or some fiber, but close clinical examination by physicians does not reveal evidence to support this assertion. These people are often treated with antipsychotic medications.

2.2.13 Itch from Head to Toe

Localized Itch

Many forms of itch (many of which have been discussed earlier) are specific to certain body areas. Here we will detail types of itch affecting different parts of the body (progressing from top to bottom).

Scalp Itch The scalp is a very itchy area of the body. It is associated with inflammatory skin diseases such as seborrheic dermatitis (dandruff), psoriasis, and hair disorders such as the scarring alopecias (hair loss disorders) and lichen planus. Finally, significant itch in the scalp can also occur as a consequence of nerve fiber damage (e.g., postherpetic neuralgia or diabetic neuropathy).

Arm and Hand Itch As discussed earlier, brachioradial pruritus is a form of localized itch that affects the arms. Liver disease also often first appears as itch in the palms before generalizing to other parts of the body.

Genital Itch A common cause of genital itch in both sexes is allergic and irritant contact dermatitis (to underwear, for example), which is associated with a strong itching and burning sensation. Frictional dermatitis can also cause itch through excessive friction between skin surfaces (more commonly seen in obese individuals).

In addition, common dermatologic conditions including both atopic dermatitis and psoriasis can specifically affect the groin and genital regions. Finally, infectious diseases can also cause significant itch and include the following: candidiasis, herpes, scabies, and chlamydia. Lichen simplex chronicus is another cause of genital itch in both men and women.

Genital itch could also be due to nerve fiber damage in the sacral region of the spinal cord and causes chronic scratching and rubbing of the skin (resulting in thickening of the skin surface in this area). It is important to also mention here that the genital area is extremely sensitive due to abundant nerve fibers in the region. For this reason, specific treatments for genital itch include anesthetic lotions, which provide a numbing effect.

Leg Itch Itch (along with pain and burning sensations) in the legs has been associated with **chronic venous insufficiency**, a very common medical condition in the population that involves the pooling of blood in the veins of the legs when the valves within the veins are not working properly.

Another cause of itch in the legs is **lichen amyloidosis**, a condition characterized by small round lesions on the legs due to deposits of a protein called amyloid in the skin. This condition typically has an increased prevalence in those with Asian or Latin American ethnicities.

3. Treating Your Itch

The term "chronic" in chronic pruritus not only describes the length of time for which it has occurred prior to seeking help but also reflects the long-term nature of its associated conditions. Like other chronic diseases, such as diabetes and asthma, there isn't a single "cure" for itch; rather, managing and minimizing itch requires finding the right treatment regimen for every individual and often requires both trial and error and treating the condition from several angles at once (for example, treating the underlying condition as well as the itch). Luckily, an increasing number of effective treatment options are available due to advances in our understanding of why itch occurs in different conditions and the subsequent development of new drugs. Now, more than ever before, living without itch is a real possibility. In this section, we will discuss all the ways we can make this possibility a reality.

3.1 Treating Itch without Medications

For all patients suffering from chronic pruritus regardless of etiology, proper skin hygiene and elimination of potential itch triggers are key for preventing and decreasing itch.

Frequent skin moisturization (to reduce dryness), avoidance of extreme temperatures, and reducing stress are just some examples of key factors that should be priorities in any anti-itch routine. In this section, we will discuss some tips and steps that you can complete on a daily basis to help you minimize, and perhaps even eliminate, itch.

3.1.1 Moisturization

Dry skin (xerosis; discussed in chapter 2.2.1) is a component of many conditions that produce itch but is also capable of producing or exacerbating itch on its own. Moisturization is the main way to both prevent and minimize dry skin. Moisturizers, such as emollients and barrier creams, are over-the-counter agents whose application should be an important part of any daily routine.

Composed of mixtures of chemical agents, including artificial or natural oils, moisturizers make skin softer by increasing and maintaining its water content. Maintaining and strengthening the skin barrier is important as it can protect internal entities (such as nerves and immune cells) from coming into contact with itchy substances or external factors that can induce itch. Different classes of moisturizers, such as ointments, creams, and lotions, have different capacities for doing this based on their ratio of oil to water.

Greatest oil/water ratio, in decreasing order:

Ointments: Excellent at keeping the skin moisturized, but can be greasy.

Creams: About 1:1 oil/water. A happy medium.

Lotions: Thinnest formulation, which makes application efficient (can comfortably put on clothes quickly after application), but not as effective as creams and ointments in moisturizing because the greater water component makes it evaporate quickly, prior to skin absorption.

Applying moisturizer is a fairly simple task, as moisturizers can be applied to both healthy and itchy skin several times a day with minimal risk. As damp skin has been shown to better absorb moisturizer, it is recommended to moisturize quickly (within a few minutes) after bathing.

Selecting a moisturizer should take into account the desired/needed level of moisturization (ointments vs. creams vs. lotions), ingredients (look for ingredients such as glycerin and hyaluronic acid!), fragrances (choosing a nonfragranced moisturizer is always a smart option, as these can be potential allergens/irritants!), and accessibility (ability to purchase in person vs. online, price, etc.). There are also numerous over-the-counter moisturizing products with anti-itch properties, often containing antipruritic ingredients like pramoxine, menthol, or calamine. In addition, a moisturizer containing SPF is a great way to save a step in your routine, as broad-spectrum SPF 30+ sunscreen application should be a mandatory part of EVERY daily routine. The best moisturizer, however, is one that you will use consistently! So, choose the potency, consistency, and formulation that fits best into your daily routine.

3.1.2 Bathing

Bathing is an important part of every daily routine for many reasons, but did you know some of your bathing habits may actually be exacerbating your itch? Here are some tips for ensuring your bathing keeps you both clean and, hopefully, itch-free:

- Use of **gentle cleansers** while bathing is recommended. A gentle cleanser is one that includes the following:
  - Has a minimal number of excess ingredients (such as fragrances or color).
  - Has a **low pH** to help maintain the skin's naturally **acidic** pH of 4.5–6. Many cleansers on the market today have an average pH of 9 or greater! A high pH like this has been associated with greater itch due to increased activity of *proteases* in the skin (see chapter 1.3).
  - Is typically **soap free** and instead made from synthetic detergents, which are typically gentler than soaps.
  - **Liquid soaps are recommended over bar soaps** as they often meet more of these criteria.
- Showers and baths should ideally be **lukewarm** and **limited in time** to prevent heat from evaporating skin moisture and irritating skin further. So no more daily shower concerts (try to keep it to one song only, OK?)!
- Patting the skin dry with a towel is preferred. Do not scrub the skin harshly with a towel after showering or bathing. This may irritate and/or break the skin and cause increased water loss.
- After taking a shower or bath, apply any prescription medications (such as topical corticosteroids) to your skin before applying moisturizers.

In addition to your regular bathing, which is sufficient, some "specialty baths" may also be helpful in soothing itchy and irritated skin. One example of this is an **oatmeal bath**, which consists of about ¼ to ¾ cup of oatmeal (ground into small pieces with a spoon) added to a full bathtub of water. Alternatively, there are several bath products containing oatmeal that you can purchase on the shelves of your local drug store. Studies have shown that oatmeal contains anti-inflammatory mediators that help decrease skin inflammation, and so, these baths can be helpful up to once a day.

3.1.3 Clothing

Wool and certain artificial fibers (nylon and polyester) can irritate the skin, activate nerve fibers, and induce itch. With this in mind, new garments have been developed that have less friction and form a protective layer around the skin. These garments help to block outside signals that trigger nerve fibers in the skin (including irritating clothing and sweat). Whenever possible, opt for clothing made with less-irritating fabrics, such as **cotton** and **silk**.

3.1.4 Stress

It has been long known that the sensation of itch is related to your state of mind, but recent research has provided more specific insight into how and why this might occur. Both stress and itch have been shown to activate similar pathways in the brain, such as the limbic system and periaqueductal gray (brain areas associated with emotions), as well as the sympathetic nervous system (your "fight-or-flight" response). Activation of these areas has, in turn, been shown to have downstream effects on the mediators of itch within the immune and nervous systems (see chapter 1). It seems that this relationship is reciprocal, with stress being able to produce or aggravate itch and itch being able to induce or increase stress.

As such, minimizing stress through various actions can be a useful tool within your chronic itch prevention and treatment toolbox. These actions can range from routinely engaging in yoga or meditation to eliminating external stressors from your daily life to seeking professional help to effectively manage any psychiatric or mental health problems. Acupuncture may also be an effective tool to help minimize stress and decrease itch (see chapter 3.4). More ideas to minimize stress to manage itch can be found in chapter 3.6.

3.1.5 Stop the Scratching!

We know that this is much easier said than done, especially if scratching provides you with immediate pleasure or relief. But, as previously discussed, scratching only increases itch in the long term and throws you deeper into that itch–scratch cycle. Stopping scratching will be difficult at first, but we promise that the pleasure and relief you'll feel long term when you no longer feel the need to scratch will be worth it. Here are a few tips to help you break the habit:

- **Keep fingernails short**. That way, when scratching does occur, there will be less damage to the skin barrier and perhaps even less pleasure felt.
- If your itch is localized, try **occluding (covering) the area** with a moisturizer and dressing (bandage) to prevent access for scratching.

- When you feel the urge to scratch, **pat the area** instead—it may give you the same nerve stimulation without the skin barrier damage.
- For children, you can implement a point/reward system: every time they verbalize itchiness but do not scratch, they earn a point toward a reward (such as pizza for dinner or a toy they want!). It's up to you whether you deduct points for catching them scratching.
- Using psychological methods may also help to break the cycle (see chapter 3.6).

3.2 Topical Treatments for Itch

Topical treatments are those that are applied directly to the skin. These are typically most effective for itch that is localized to a specific region of the body. They may also be used for "spot treatment" of the most severe areas of skin disease for those on systemic therapy (pills, injections). Topical treatments typically have less side effects than systemic therapies, so your doctor may prefer to try them first.

3.2.1 Cooling Agents

Menthol has been used for centuries to treat itch and is effective at reducing itch through a cooling effect on the skin. It works through activating specific transient receptor potential (TRP) channels on nerve fibers and keratinocytes that are cold-sensitive. Menthol has also been reported to work on the **kappa-opioid receptor** system. For people who notice that their itch is improved by a cold shower or application of an ice cube, such as **neuropathic itch**, this medication may be helpful. Other cooling agents that are available (and are often combined with other antipruritic therapies) include camphor and calamine lotion.

3.2.2 Topical Anesthetics

Topical anesthetics that have been found to have anti-itch effects include pramoxine, prilocaine, lidocaine, and polidocanol. These agents work by blocking the transmission of nerve impulses. Pramoxine 1% is effective in treating many different types of itch. In particular, it is effective at reducing itch in facial and genital areas, as well as treating neuropathic itch. In addition, a pramoxine-based anti-itch lotion has shown efficacy in treating pruritus in adults who are undergoing hemodialysis. Polidocanol is another topical agent that is not currently available in the United States. A combination of 3% polidocanol and 5% urea significantly reduced itch in people with atopic dermatitis, contact dermatitis, and psoriasis. As discussed in the moisturization section of the previous chapter, some moisturizers contain these ingredients and are labeled "anti-itch." Choosing these might be a good way to save time in your daily routine and achieve maximal itch relief, alongside other treatments.

Additionally, combination **topical ketamine-amitriptyline-lidocaine (TKAL)** has been shown to be very successful in treating itch in both prurigo nodularis and neuropathic itch. This type of combination formula can be prescribed by your doctor, often through a specialty compounding pharmacy.

Topical **capsaicin** (the active ingredient of chili peppers) causes the release of *substance P*, a stress-associated neuropeptide that is known to play a role in itch. While this may seem counterintuitive, capsaicin works to relieve itch by proactively *depleting* the substance P stored within your cells. Capsaicin also is known to bind to the **transient receptor potential vanilloid 1** (TRPV1), a heat-sensitive receptor on neurons and keratinocytes. Therefore, initial application of capsaicin causes a transient burning sensation. This adverse effect, however, typically resolves after this medicine is used for a few days or alongside a topical anesthetic.

Capsaicin is especially effective at reducing itch that originates from nerve fibers (neuropathic itch), including postherpetic itch, brachioradial pruritus, and notalgia paresthetica (see chapter 2.2.6). In addition, capsaicin is effective at reducing itch associated with psoriasis and chronic kidney disease. Caution should be used: avoid applying capsaicin to genital and mucosal areas, as it causes a stinging sensation.

3.2.3 Topical Antihistamines

Topical antihistamines may be useful for some acute itchy conditions, including bug bites and hives, but as most chronically itchy conditions act through nonhistaminergic pathways (see chapter 1.3), they have limited use in chronic pruritus. Topical **doxepin**, an antidepressant with antihistaminergic effects, however, has been found effective in treating pruritus in inflammatory skin diseases with side effects of drowsiness and contact dermatitis that sometimes limit its use.

3.2.4 Topical Corticosteroids

Topical corticosteroids are anti-inflammatory creams and ointments. They are often the first agents prescribed by dermatologists for people suffering from itch associated with inflammatory skin diseases such as atopic dermatitis, psoriasis, contact dermatitis, and lichen planus (see chapter 2.2.2). Topical corticosteroids directly treat inflammation (often appearing as the rash) as opposed to treating the underlying cause of itch. Therefore, topical corticosteroids do not directly decrease itch but rather indirectly decrease the sensation of itch by reducing inflammation of the skin. If there is no inflammation present (such as itch of neuropathic, systemic, psychogenic, or unknown etiologies), these medications have minimal value.

Topical corticosteroids come in several different potencies and vehicles (including creams, ointments, gels, sprays, and lotions). Table 3.1 ranks some of the most commonly prescribed steroids in order of potency. It is good practice for your doctor to prescribe the **least-potent steroid** that will effectively treat your condition at its current severity to minimize the side effects of topical steroids (most prominently, skin thinning). You may also be prescribed several steroids at once to keep at home in preparation for flaring disease of different severities. Using table 3.1 as a reference can help *you* decide what is needed at a given time.

When using topical steroids, it is important to apply them correctly in order to get the maximal benefit and minimal risk for side effects. For many people, the most challenging aspect of this is determining how much to

Table 3.1 Commonly Prescribed Topical Steroids in Order of Potency

Class	Generic drug names
I (very high potency)	Clobetasol propionate 0.05% (cream and ointment)
II (high potency)	Betamethasone dipropionate 0.05% (ointment) Desoximetasone 0.25% (cream) Fluocinonide 0.05% (cream and ointment) Mometasone furoate 0.1% (ointment)
III	Betamethasone dipropionate 0.05% (cream) Betamethasone valerate 0.1% (ointment) Fluticasone propionate 0.005% (ointment)
IV (mid-potency)	Fluocinolone acetonide 0.025% (ointment) Mometasone furoate 0.1% (cream) Triamcinolone acetonide 0.1% (cream)
V	Betamethasone valerate 0.1% (cream) Fluocinolone acetonide 0.025% (cream) Fluticasone propionate 0.05% (cream)
VI (low potency)	Alclometasone dipropionate 0.05% (ointment) Clobetasone butyrate 0.05% (Cream) Desonide 0.05% (cream and ointment)
VII	Hydrocortisone (acetate) 1% (cream and ointment) Hydrocortisone aceponate 0.127% (cream)

apply at a given time. While the answer to this question is complex and based on the extent of disease and the potency of the corticosteroid, the **fingertip rule** (see chapter 3.5) is typically a good rule to follow when using a mild to medium topical corticosteroid.

If you are applying another cream, such as a moisturizer, care should be taken to apply these about 15–30 minutes apart to allow for maximal absorption of both. The moisturizer should always be applied first.

For people suffering from atopic dermatitis, psoriasis, and other inflammatory itchy disorders, **wet pajamas** (also known as wet wrap therapy) can be an extremely useful tool in alleviating itch (see "Practical Nursing Tips" below).

3.2.5 Topical Calcineurin Inhibitors

Tacrolimus and pimecrolimus are two non-steroid-based anti-inflammatory medications known as *calcineurin inhibitors* (brand names Elidel and Protopic). These drugs are immunomodulating agents, meaning that they work similarly to corticosteroids in suppressing inflammation. On the molecular level, these drugs work on TRPV1 (transient receptor potential vanilloid 1) ion channels on neurons. These drugs have been effective in reducing itch associated with atopic dermatitis, prurigo nodularis, and lichen sclerosus, and they are also typically used for facial, hand, and anogenital itch. These agents are particularly useful for the face and armpits, areas where topical corticosteroids are traditionally not used due to concern for **skin atrophy**. A commonly encountered side

effect from these drugs is a temporary burning or stinging sensation.

3.2.6 Topical PDE-4 Inhibitors

Phosphodiesterase-4 (PDE-4) is an enzyme that increases
the production of inflammatory cytokines (see chapter 1.3).
Inhibiting this enzyme has anti-inflammatory effects and
has been shown to reduce itch. **Crisaborole**, a topical PDE-4
inhibitor that is approved for treating atopic dermatitis, has
been shown to decrease itch intensity in as little as a few
days. More recently, a new more potent PDE-4 inhibitor,
Roflumilast, has shown to be effective in cases of localized
itch such as seborrheic dermatitis, eczema, and psoriasis.

3.2.7 Topical JAK-STAT Inhibitors

The role of the Janus kinase (JAK)/STAT pathway in itch
is an emerging field of research with great promise for
treating many inflammatory itchy conditions. The JAK/
STAT pathway has been shown to broadly dysregulate
immune responses and increase production of inflammatory cytokines; therefore, inhibiting this pathway is
anti-inflammatory. Topical **ruxolitinib (Opzelura)** was
approved in the US for the treatment of atopic dermatitis.
Topical compounded tofacitinib has been shown to
effectively decrease itch in conditions like atopic dermatitis and psoriasis and prurigo nodularis. Topical **delgoci-
tinib** was recently approved in Japan for the treatment of
pruritus in atopic dermatitis and has been shown to be
both effective and well tolerated.

3.2.8 Topical Cannabinoids

The rationale for using topical **cannabinoids** (such as cannabidiol [CBD] and tetrahydrocannabinol [THC]) in the treatment of itch came with the finding that cannabinoid **receptors** are expressed on **keratinocytes (skin cells)**, **mast cells**, and nerve fibers. Lotions and ointments including CBD, most of which can be bought over the counter, have been shown to reduce itch in atopic dermatitis. Generally, CBD-containing substances are considered safe when applied topically and do not have the psychoactive effects of substances that contain THC (the main psychoactive substance in marijuana). N-palmitoylethanolamine is also a medication that stimulates cannabinoid receptors and has been incorporated into creams; it has been shown to reduce itch associated with atopic dermatitis and chronic kidney disease.

Do You Want to Learn More?

See online supplement for an interactive graphic on medications that work on the skin, nerves, spinal cord, and brain.

3.3 Systemic Treatments for Itch

Systemic therapies are those that travel through the bloodstream and reach your skin and nerves all over the body. As such, these treatments are best for people with generalized itch or localized itch that is unresponsive to topical therapies.

3.3.1 Antihistamines

Oral antihistamines have long been one of the first-line treatments for itch. As their name suggests, antihistamines work through blocking the action of histamine. Thus, antihistamines can be effective in disorders where histamine triggers itch (for example, chronic urticaria or hives).

There are several types of antihistamines, which can be divided into sedating and nonsedating. Sedating antihistamines, like hydroxyzine and diphenhydramine, can be useful for itch that is most severe at night. Nonsedating antihistamines, like cetirizine, desloratadine, loratadine, and levocetirizine, may be more helpful for daytime itch and are especially useful at targeting diseases in which histamine is an important component of the itch (for example, urticaria, drug-related itch, and chronic insect bites). As most forms of chronic itch, however, are produced through a nonhistaminergic pathway (see chapter 1.3), nonsedating antihistamines are of limited efficacy in chronic itch. It should also be noted that the long-term use of sedating antihistamines has been found to have some association with the development of dementia and is thus not recommended.

3.3.2 Neuroactive Medications

Neuroactive medications act on your nervous system! These include medications like gabapentin and pregabalin—medications that have traditionally been referred to as "antiseizure medications" but have many uses beyond the treatment of seizures. These medications have been shown to be effective at controlling pain in people with chronic pain syndromes in addition to chronic itch.

While how they work isn't precisely known, they are thought to decrease the processing of itchy stimuli through the nerves to the brain. In a sense, they "quiet" your nerves so that you feel less itchy. As such, they are especially effective in forms of neuropathic itch (see chapter 2.2.6), like postherpetic itch, brachioradial pruritus, and notalgia paresthetica. In addition, these medications have been shown to be effective in people suffering from cutaneous lymphomas, chronic kidney disease (when used after each dialysis session), and even chronic pruritus of unknown origin. These drugs are particularly useful for those whose itch is exacerbated at nighttime, as drowsiness can be a common side effect. Other common side effects include weight gain, lower limb swelling, blurry vision, and constipation. In order to reduce these adverse effects and improve tolerability, these drugs need to be gradually increased in dose (titration). Additionally, when stopping these medications, it is important to gradually decrease or wean the dose prior to ceasing use completely to avoid withdrawal symptoms.

3.3.3 Antidepressants

We previously discussed the interrelationship between itch, the brain, and the psyche. This connection explains why antidepressants have been shown to be effective in reducing itch in many people. It is important to note that all antidepressants usually take about two to four weeks to get into a person's system before a significant benefit can be seen. There are several types of antidepressants on the market, but those that are useful in treating chronic itch can be generally classified into two categories based on neurotransmitter(s) they increase within the brain.

1. *Antidepressants that increase the amount of norepinephrine and serotonin in the brain.* Mirtazapine increases the amount of both norepinephrine and serotonin in the brain. For patients with chronic itch that exacerbates at nighttime, mirtazapine may be an especially effective drug since it can improve mood and enhance sleep. One of the side effects of mirtazapine is that it may stimulate your appetite (and cause weight gain); another side effect is drowsiness. Usually low doses of this drug (15 mg or less) work for itch, while higher doses are more useful for depression and anxiety.

2. *Antidepressants that increase the amount of serotonin in the brain (aka selective serotonin reuptake inhibitors, or SSRIs).* These drugs specifically increase primarily the amount of serotonin in the brain and include fluoxetine (Prozac), fluvoxamine, paroxetine, and sertraline. These can be useful in those with a comorbid depression or anxiety diagnosis, or those who experience such symptoms as a result of their itch. Low-dose sertraline, in particular, is also useful for cholestatic pruritus.

3.3.4 Opioid Stimulators and Blockers

Opioids, such as morphine, have been known for some time to be extremely important in blocking pain transmission; they have also been shown to worsen itch. Recently, imbalances in opioids naturally found in the body have been implicated in the pathophysiology of itch. Research has revealed the importance of subgroups of **opioid receptors** in the brain, including mu and kappa opioids. Specifically, there seems to be an inverse relationship present: stimulation of the mu-opioid receptor *increases* itch and stimulation of the kappa-opioid receptor *decreases* itch. As such, drugs that block the mu-opioid receptor and/or activate the kappa-opioid receptor have the capability to decrease itch.

Did You Know?

Morphine and other common opioid medications reduce pain while conversely having the potential effect of exacerbating itch. This itch is caused by stimulation of the mu-opioid receptors, which are located in the brain, spinal cord, and various organs. These receptors can be blocked by mu-opioid receptor blockers, such as naltrexone.

Mu-Opioid Receptor Blockers
Naltrexone, the most commonly prescribed mu-opioid receptor blocker in chronic itch, has been shown to reduce itch in people with liver disease, chronic kidney

disease, atopic dermatitis, and those suffering from postburn itch. Possible side effects include nausea, vomiting, and drowsiness. It is important that those taking other opioid drugs for pain notify their doctor before taking this medication, as it will reverse the analgesic effect and potentially precipitate opioid withdrawal.

Combination Mu-Opioid Receptor Blockers/Kappa-Opioid Receptor Stimulators

Butorphanol is a currently available drug that both stimulates and blocks the kappa- and mu- opioid receptors, respectively. It is given intranasally and effective in the treatment of chronic refractory itch in people whose itch is the result of inflammatory skin diseases and systemic conditions. It is important to note that this is one of the last-line treatments for itch and considered a controlled substance by the FDA.

Kappa-Opioid Receptor Stimulators

Difelikefalin is a kappa-opioid receptor stimulator that has been approved for chronic kidney disease itch and is administered via a needle to the vein. Nalfurafine, which is currently available only in Japan, is approved for the treatment of chronic kidney disease and liver-associated pruritus.

3.3.5 Substance P and NK-1 Inhibitors

Substance P and its receptor neurokinin 1 (NK-1) are known mediators of itch that are located throughout the skin and central nervous system. **Aprepitant**, an NK-1 blocker used to treat chemotherapy-induced nausea, has previously been successful in treating intractable itch due to prurigo nodularis and cutaneous T-cell lymphoma (CTCL); however, its expensive price tag and numerous interactions with other drugs have limited its practicality and use.

In recent years, newer NK-1 antagonists have undergone clinical trials but have shown limited promise. While **serlopitant** displayed some efficacy in treating severe itch in psoriasis, it was found less efficacious in treating itch associated with prurigo nodularis or chronic pruritus of unknown origin (CPUO). **Tradipitant**, another NK-1 inhibitor, was similarly ineffective in treating itch in atopic dermatitis. These disappointing results have somewhat hampered development of drugs targeting this pathway.

3.3.6 Cannabinoids

While the role of cannabinoids within our immune system and the itch pathways is still not fully understood, it seems that activation of specific cannabinoid receptors within the skin and nervous system can help relieve both pain and itch. **Dronabinol**, a synthetic form of delta-9-tetrahydrocannabinol, has specifically been shown to reduce itching in both cholestatic and neuropathic itch. This relief often has a rapid onset but is short-lasting. Larger, controlled trials are still necessary to understand the true efficacy and safety of cannabinoids in the treatment of itch.

3.3.7 Drugs That Work on the Immune System

Oral Corticosteroids

These are drugs that reduce the amount of inflammation present in the body. They have no direct anti-itch
effect. They are particularly effective for calming severe
flares of inflammatory itchy conditions (typically associated with rash) that are not infectious. These are not a
long-term solution, however, as prolonged use of these
medications can cause adverse side effects (increased
susceptibility to disease, Cushing syndrome, bone frac-
tures, and diabetes).

Biologics

Biologics are substances that are made from living
organisms that stop inflammation. **Dupilumab** is a newer
treatment approved for atopic dermatitis that specifically
targets cytokines IL-4 and IL-13 that are important in
atopic dermatitis. It blocks the IL-4 receptor, which, in
turn, blocks the actions of the IL-4 cytokine. It has been
shown to have dramatic, anti-itch effects that begin as
early as the first week of treatment. This success has
caused it to quickly become the first-line treatment for
many patients with moderate to severe eczema. In recent
years, however, we have begun to see that it may also be
efficacious in other itchy conditions. Recently, dupilumab
has been approved in the US for the treatment of prurigo
nodularis. Additionally, it has been used off-label in
treating chronic pruritus of unknown origin, bullous
pemphigoid, and chronic urticaria. Clinical trials are
currently under way to test its efficacy and safety in
several of these conditions. Due to the drug's relative

safety and minor side effects (conjunctivitis and injection site reactions) in combination with the promising results we've seen thus far, we expect the role of dupilumab in the treatment of chronic pruritus to continue to increase in the coming years.

In addition to dupilumab, tralokinumab, a monoclonal antibody against IL-13, has been approved for atopic eczema. Lebrikizumab, another monoclonal antibody against IL-13, has shown promising results in clinical trials for reducing itch in atopic dermatitis but has not yet been approved. Nemolizumab, which targets the itchy cytokine IL-31, has also shown great promise in clinical trials for atopic dermatitis as well as prurigo nodularis and is expecting approval. Omalizumab is a drug inhibiting binding antibody immunoglobulin E (IgE) that causes chronic urticaria.

JAK/STAT Inhibitors

As discussed in the previous chapter, the role of the Janus kinase (JAK)/STAT pathway in itch is an emerging field of research with great promise for treating many inflammatory itchy conditions. The JAK/STAT pathway has been shown to broadly affect immune responses and increase production of inflammatory cytokines; therefore, inhibiting this pathway is anti-inflammatory. Recently, several drugs that inhibit aspects of this pathway have been approved for the treatment of several itchy conditions. For example, **abrocitinib (Cibinqo)** was approved for moderate to severe atopic dermatitis in adults. **Upadacitinib (Rinvoq)** has been approved for the treatment of moderate to severe atopic dermatitis in adults and children 12 years and older whose disease did not respond or is not controlled with other medications. These drugs show a rapid and robust anti-itch effect.

Baricitinib was recently approved for the treatment of severe alopecia areata (an autoimmune hair loss condition that may sometimes itch) and has been approved in Europe for severe atopic dermatitis. **Upadacitinib** and **tofacitinib** have been approved for the treatment of psoriatic arthritis but may have impacts on the associated psoriatic skin disease and itch as well. **Deucravacitinib**, a tyrosine kinase 2 (TYK2) inhibitor (**SOTYKTU**), an enzyme part of this same JAK/STAT pathway, has been recently approved for the treatment of psoriasis. The broad anti-inflammatory effects of these drugs may make them useful in a variety of other inflammatory response-derived itchy diseases, and studies investigating their efficacy are ongoing.

Drugs Targeting Interleukin 17 and 23 Inhibitors
Drugs for treatment of psoriasis-blocking interleukin 17 and interleukin 23, such as secukinumab (Cosentyx), ixekizumab (Taltz), and brodalumab (Siliq), and drugs inhibiting IL-23, such as guselkumab (Tremfaya), risanki-zumab (Skyrizi), and tildrakizumab (Ilumya), have all shown anti-itch effects in psoriatic patients.

Drugs Targeting Bruton Tyrosine Kinase Receptors
Bruton tyrosine kinase (BTK) inhibitors are a new class of selective drugs that show promising anti-itch effect in chronic spontaneous urticaria (CSU). Remibrutinib, which showed significant anti-itch effect and a good safety

profile, is under FDA approval for CSU that is unresponsive to antihistamines.

Immunosuppressants

Cyclosporine, Azathioprine, and Mycophenolate Mofetil are effective at suppressing an overactive immune system. They can have efficacy in controlling itch associated with inflammatory conditions; however, for many of these conditions, they are no longer considered first-line treatments due to newer, more targeted treatments entering the market. These agents are recommended for short-term use in the treatment of atopic dermatitis and prurigo nodularis in people whose symptoms have failed to respond to other therapies. In addition, cyclosporine is a useful agent in those with chronic spontaneous urticaria.

While taking these agents, it is important that patients are monitored carefully for adverse effects. Patients on azathioprine should have lab work done regularly to check blood counts and liver enzymes for abnormalities. Cyclosporine has been associated with high blood pressure and kidney dysfunction that requires careful monthly monitoring of kidney function. Mycophenolate mofetil may cause diarrhea and nausea.

Methotrexate

Methotrexate is an oral anticancer drug that can also be used to suppress the immune system in low doses in people who have atopic dermatitis, psoriasis, prurigo nodularis, and cutaneous lymphoma. It has also been shown to be effective in patients with chronic pruritus of unknown origin, especially those with chronic pruritus of aging.

This drug interacts with the immune system by decreasing activity of the immune system. In some patients, this drug lowers the white blood cell count, especially in the first weeks after it is given. A low white blood cell count increases the chance of getting a serious infection. This drug can also cause liver toxicity, especially in those who drink alcohol regularly or have a fatty liver. Therefore, regular monitoring of blood counts and liver function is required when patients are taking methotrexate. It is also important to note that methotrexate can cause serious birth defects and should never be taken by a patient who is pregnant or planning to become pregnant.

Thalidomide

Thalidomide is an oral agent that has the effect of decreasing the overactivity of the immune system as well as the nervous system. It should be one of the last-line treatments for itch associated with chronic prurigo nodularis, kidney disease, or cutaneous T-cell lymphoma. Thalidomide has significant potential side effects, especially birth defects in offspring of women of childbearing age (it is not to be used at all during pregnancy), blood clots, peripheral nerve fiber damage, and drowsiness. It is given by dermatologists who have a special license to administer this drug and requires monthly visits to monitor its side effects.

3.3.8 Phototherapy

Phototherapy can be helpful in the treatment of many itchy conditions (ranging from common dermatologic conditions such as atopic dermatitis and psoriasis to itch associated with systemic conditions including chronic kidney or liver disease and itch associated with HIV). The different forms of phototherapy include both broadband and narrowband ultraviolet B (UVB) and ultraviolet A (UVA). These agents can be used individually, in combination with one another, or with a compound known as psoralen that can be ingested orally or applied topically. While the exact mechanism is unknown for how phototherapy can decrease itch, it has been suggested that it results in the chemical modification of itch-producing factors.

3.4 Complementary and Alternative Treatments for Itch

Acknowledgment: Dr. Peter Lio

In addition to the typical over-the-counter and pharmacologic treatments recommended by your physicians, there are also numerous other techniques and products that may be useful as part of your "anti-itch" regimen. **Complementary medicines** are those that are used in conjunction with conventional medicine, whereas the term "alternative" refers to those that are used in place of conventional medicine. Many of these treatments and techniques aim to integrate physical, psychological, and nutritional health by using traditional medicinal techniques, botanical products, and nutritional supplementation.

In this chapter, we will discuss some of the complementary and alternative medicines (CAMs) that may help decrease itch. It is important to note that most CAMs have not been as rigorously studied as conventional medicines and lack regulatory agencies that control procedure certifications and ingredients. Therefore, prior to beginning any of these therapies, we recommend consulting with your physician.

3.4.1 Hydrogels and Bleach

There has been a lot of discussion about dilute bleach baths for atopic dermatitis. Similar to the levels of chlorine in a swimming pool, this relatively gentle treatment has been shown to have both anti-inflammatory and anti-itch effects. There are now over-the-counter formulations that aim to be like "a dilute bleach bath in a bottle," and one form of this is with a stabilized hydrogel. Hydrogels are gels composed of hypochlorous acid or sodium hypochlorite (the active part of bleach) that have been compared to antihistamines and steroids in terms of their itch-reducing ability. It has been hypothesized that they function as anti-inflammatory agents and may also decrease water loss from the skin, helping to improve the skin barrier in patients with atopic dermatitis. They come in convenient spray bottles, and they are relatively safe and fairly inexpensive. In addition to the potential for anti-itch effects, there may be some antibacterial effect, in addition to the cooling sensation when a light gel is applied to the skin. All of these factors may work to help with itching. When conventional therapies have not shown great improvement in itch, these may serve as a safe alternative when used with moisturizers, as they have been noted to sometimes cause skin dryness.

3.4.2 Botanicals

The application of different oils to the skin (and their addition to many moisturizers available for over-the-counter purchase) is a popular alternative therapy in skin conditions with dry skin and impaired barrier function. While **olive oil** is a common and popular addition, it has actually been shown to damage the skin barrier through reducing the integrity of the stratum corneum. Conversely, **sunflower seed oil** and **virgin coconut oil** have been shown to improve the skin barrier and produce anti-inflammatory effects. **Evening primrose oil** and **borage oil** may also facilitate skin barrier repair and have anti-inflammatory properties, although its supporting data are more limited.

Remarkably, one small study in patients with itch associated with chronic kidney disease showed significant improvement in itch after seven minutes of hand massage with a mixture of natural oils including lavender, mint, and tea tree oil at a 5% concentration.

While generally safe, it is possible to be allergic to plant-based oils, so it is always advisable to try a small area of skin first before applying broadly. Additionally, most of the natural oils are not ideal moisturizer replacements and may be better used in addition to more conventional moisturizers to help protect the skin.

Cannabinoids are a large category of chemicals that are found in the hemp plant and the marijuana plant. While medical marijuana is helpful for certain conditions, one specific molecule called cannabidiol (CBD) is being studied for its potential to help with itch and inflammation. Unlike marijuana, CBD has no psychoactive effects and when applied topically does not appear to get absorbed enough to cause any issues with the brain or rest of the body. There is still much to learn about this group of compounds, however, and it is difficult to know if a given product will be of sufficient quality at this point.

3.4.3 Acupressure and Acupuncture

Acupressure and acupuncture are two similar techniques that originate from Asia and are a mainstay in several traditional medicine systems. **Acupuncture**, the more well-known technique of the two, involves the insertion of thin needles into specific body points to clear blockages at "meridians" that allow life energy to flow properly through-out the body. While the list of claimed benefits of this procedure is incredibly large and frequently debated, several studies have shown that it may decrease itch. There are also

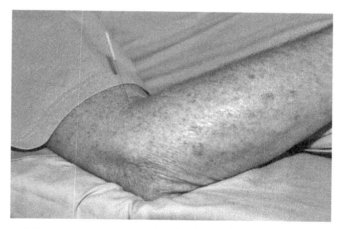

Figure 3.1   Acupuncture point for itch: Chinese medicine believes there is a distribution network that relates to internal organs called the meridian system. The large intestine meridian L11 in the elbow was found to be an effective site for treating itch. Author photo.

studies, though, that show no effect of any symptom improvement. Adverse effects of acupuncture are fortunately rare, but infection, nerve injury, hemorrhage, skin necrosis, and collapsed lung have been reported, so caution is advised, and working with a reputable practitioner is critical.

Acupressure is a similar technique to acupuncture that aims to improve fatigue, pain, and itch. Instead of using needles, acupressure utilizes physical pressure applied to specific body points, making it a safer alternative with rare adverse effects. Several studies have been conducted in recent years that show it may be a safe and helpful adjunctive treatment in patients with atopic dermatitis and the itch associated with chronic kidney disease, with similar benefits to acupuncture. Both of these modalities require finding a suitable practitioner, going for repeated visits, and generally paying out of pocket, so they may not be a good fit for everyone.

3.4.4 Nutritional Supplements

While not yet rigorously studied, several nutritional supplements have been noted to decrease itch. **Quercetin** is a plant-derived flavonoid with anti-inflammatory and antioxidant properties that has been noted in small studies to reduce itch in prurigo nodularis without any major side effects noted to date. **N-acetyl cysteine (NAC)** has been noted in several small studies to decrease anxiety, which may help to decrease scratching and picking in a variety of itchy conditions; however, side effects include nausea and vomiting, urticaria, and rash. Consult with your physician prior to starting NAC, as it should be avoided in patients with a tendency to develop anaphylactic reactions, fluid overload, or gastrointestinal ulcers.

Impatiens balsamina **L** (also known as spotted snapweed, touch-me-not, and garden balsam) is a long-used Japanese folk remedy for itching that is similar to henna and can be taken orally in extract form. It has been shown to decrease scratching behavior but should be taken with caution and supervision as it can be toxic in large doses and also reduce testosterone levels at all doses. It should also be avoided in people with arthritis, gout, kidney stones, and hyperacidity.

In addition to oral supplementation, **topical vitamin B12** has been shown to improve disease symptoms, including itch, in patients with atopic dermatitis.

3.4.5 Conclusion

While evidence for the above treatments is promising, further investigation is needed to truly understand if and how they help to alleviate itch. Like all other treatment modalities discussed in this book, it is important to consult your physician prior to beginning any new treatments or management techniques to ensure safety. Therefore, finding a physician who is experienced in integrative medicine techniques and their role in skin disease management is advisable.

3.5 Practical Nursing Tips
Acknowledgment: Juan M. Gonzales, DNP, APRN

Taking a multidisciplinary approach toward managing itch can be extremely beneficial and effective. Hearing the perspectives, viewpoints, and paradigms of specialists in different fields and incorporating their knowledge into your anti-itch management plan not only allows you to personalize your care toward your own needs but also ensures you have a well-rounded and balanced approach to targeting your itch from different angles. Nurses play an important role within this multidisciplinary team, reinforcing key aspects of health promotion and disease prevention through practical education of the patient and their families. In fact, teaching by dermatology nurses about the use of topical therapy may reduce itch and disease severity in patients with atopic itch by 89%, according to some studies, and improve overall patient outcomes.

Specifically, nurses can be an extremely useful resource for understanding how to best use the pharmacologic therapies you are prescribed and incorporate them into your daily life for maximum efficacy. Below are some of my favorite tips and tricks I love to teach my patients and have found to be extremely useful in itch management:

3.5.1 The "Fingertip Rule" for Topical Steroid Application

To determine how much topical mild to moderate potency steroid is needed for a particular body region, it can be useful to follow this general rule (table 3.2). One "fingertip unit" consists of the amount of cream squeezed out from the tip of your finger to your first knuckle (see figure 3.2).

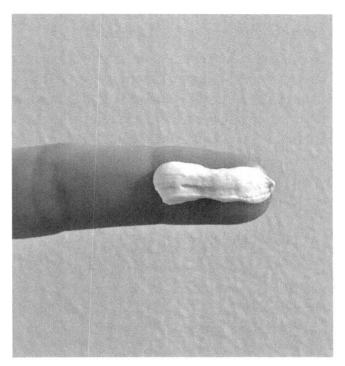

Figure 3.2   One fingertip unit of topical steroid cream.
Author photo.

Table 3.2   The Fingertip Rule for Applying Mild to Moderate Potency Topical Corticosteroids

Body region	Number of fingertip units required
Hands	1 each
Arms	3 each
Feet	2 each
Legs	6 each
Face and neck	2.5 total
Trunk, front and back	14 total
Entire body	~40 total

3.5.2 "Wet Pajama" or "Wet Wrap Therapy"

Applying your topical steroids using the "**wet pajama**" or "**wet wrap**" method can help to soften the skin by increasing moisture, prevent water loss through the skin, cool the skin, provide occlusion (which can enhance the absorption of medications), and provide a physical barrier to prevent scratching. Double-layer wet pajamas are worn during the night but can be an effective method to reduce itch during all times of the day. There are many video tutorials on the internet for how to best do this, but the basic technique is as follows:

1. Take a shower or soak yourself in a bath.
2. A moisturizing lotion, cream, or topical corticosteroid should be applied to the affected areas of the skin.
3. A wet pair of pajamas that has been soaked in water should be worn on top of the creams.
4. A dry pair of pajamas should be worn on top.
5. Now you are ready to go to sleep. You should sleep through the night. If for some reason your itch is aggravated, you can remove the dry layer of pajamas and rewet the inner layer.

Wet-layer pajamas are recommended to be used in one-week intervals.

Do You Want to Learn More?

See online supplement for a video on the double wet layer pajama treatment for relief of chronic itch.

3.5.3 Unna Boots

An Unna boot is a type of occlusive dressing that may be requested by your doctor to treat severe leg ulceration, inflammation, and itching. It is made up of a gauze soaked in zinc oxide (a compound known to improve wound healing) and potentially steroid cream, calamine lotion, or other topical therapies wrapped around your lower leg from your toes to your knee. It is then followed by an outer wrap that applies support and compression. When left in place for one to two weeks, it functions by not only improving healing of the underlying wounds but also preventing access to the damaged skin region for itching.

Once applied by the nursing staff, it is important to follow a few simple instructions to ensure that it is as effective as possible:

DO:

Keep leg elevated above the level of your heart whenever possible.

Keep it dry. Use a heavy plastic bag taped above and below the boot when showering or keep the leg completely out of the tub if taking a bath.

Continue to walk daily, if possible, to increase blood circulation to the lower leg.

Monitor your toes for any change in color (blue, white, darkening), cold temperature, swelling, or numbness.

DON'T:

Put any object into the boot or under the dressing to relieve itching.

3.5.4 Cool Your Creams!

Have you found that cooling, with an icepack, cool compress, or cold shower, helps to relieve your itch? If so, try keeping your moisturizing creams in the refrigerator! The cooling sensation on the skin from applying a refrigerated product may help calm itch and give a more soothing effect than a room temperature product. Just be sure to read the storage instructions for any product you decide to refrigerate beforehand so it doesn't diminish its efficacy.

Next time you go for your dermatology or primary care appointment, see what tips and tricks the nurses might have for you!

3.6 Psychological Management of Itch

Acknowledgment: Dr. Christina Schut

Itchy skin conditions have been associated with various psychological phenomena such as stress, anxiety, depression, and sleep disorders While there is a lack of studies investigating whether psychological factors actually cause itch or get exacerbated by it, it is reasonable to assume that both are likely to have impacts on each other and that a vicious cycle of itch and psychological factors needs to be broken by the patients.

Health professionals like dermatologists, psychiatrists, psychologists, and nurses can help to break the cycle by offering different kinds of social support. Social support can be divided into professional and nonprofessional social support. The latter is usually provided by friends or family. Nonprofessional social support can further be differentiated into emotional (e.g., being empathetic), instrumental (e.g., spending money for a new treatment or helping in the household), evaluative (i.e., supporting the opinion of the patient), and informational (e.g., giving advice or helping the patient to find evidence-based information material) support. As social support can lower the physiological and psychological stress response, it is very likely to also have effects on skin symptoms like itch.

In addition to social support, psychological interventions are useful in the management of itch when accompanied by psychological factors. In this section, we discuss some interventions that have been shown to be successful in patients with chronic pruritus. While some of the interventions mentioned below have been shown to be effective alone, a combination of different methods might be especially useful.

3.6.1 Relaxation Techniques

There are different ways of relaxing and relieving stress (e.g., meeting with friends, exercising, or doing yoga). Additionally, a few structured relaxation techniques have been shown to positively alter the physiological and psychological stress response. Progressive muscle relaxation (PMR) and autogenic training are two widely accepted relaxation trainings that can help patients with chronic itch relax. In order for either of these techniques to be successful, patients should be open to and welcoming of their success.

PMR is a form of stress-reducing, guided relaxation that effectively reduces bodily symptoms like pain and itch and improves sleep in patients with atopic dermatitis. It follows the belief of 20th-century American physician Edmund Jacobson that tension must first be experienced before true relaxation can be achieved. Thus, instructions involve selectively contracting, and subsequently relaxing, different muscle groups Engaging in this technique on a regular basis may help decrease itch intensity as well as improve sleep.

AT (autogenetic training) is another relaxation technique that is known to reduce stress and anxiety. In contrast to PMR, AT does not require physical movements by the patients—rather, it asks you to simply imagine certain things happening to your body. An AT facilitator, whether in person or in audio form, will guide the patient to focus on bodily sensations, including warmth, heaviness, and calmness, using phrases such as "your right arm is heavy" or "I feel very calm." Guided sensations can be altered depending on what feels comfortable to the patient. Maintaining a regular heartbeat and steady breath is key in this exercise.

3.6.2 Stress Relaxation

Stress is known to aggravate itch. Please refer to https://www.youtube.com/watch?v=G7sdgBMxzbE for an example of Guided Deep Muscle Relaxation techniques.

3.6.3 Mindfulness

According to Jon Kabat-Zinn, the founder of modern mindfulness, mindfulness is a certain kind of attention that involves focusing on the present moment without judging it. Mindfulness-based interventions such as Mindfulness Based Cognitive Therapy (MBCT) have been shown to increase quality of life and reduce unpleasant physical symptoms. Even though Kabat-Zinn conducted one of his first studies on the effects of mindfulness in patients with psoriasis, the next studies on the effects of mindfulness-based training in patients with chronic itch were not published until about 20 years later. New results are somewhat conflicting; studies found mindfulness-based interventions to be effective in patients with chronic itch, while others could not support these positive effects. Components of a mindfulness routine can include breathing exercises, focusing on body sensations or sounds, and can easily be incorporated into various daily activities like brushing teeth, eating, or walks .

3.6.4 Biofeedback

Biofeedback is a technique that aims to bring conscious awareness to the typically unconscious processes that occur within our bodies with the aim of learning to control physiological functions. These bodily reactions include our muscle tonus, blood flow, or temperature—all of which can be measured by various technologies and thus be reported to the patients. It has been shown that by becoming more aware of these processes, people are able to alter their bodily reactions. Even though biofeedback has been used effectively in patients with pain, the effects of biofeedback on chronic itch have not been studied comprehensively.

3.6.5 Psychotherapy

If itch occurs as part of a psychological condition or in a patient with an existing psychological disorder (anxiety, depression, ADHD, etc.), psychotherapy is a useful addition to the treatment regimen. Specific goals for psychotherapy should be agreed on by the patient and psychotherapist.

There are different kinds of psychotherapy, but when the patient with chronic itch is plagued by irrational thoughts regarding the itchy skin condition (e.g., "I will never find a partner because of my skin appearance"), **cognitive restructuring** as part of **cognitive behavioral therapy** might be helpful. In cognitive restructuring, situations in which irrational thoughts occur are first identified. Then the thought itself as well as its consequences are described by the patients. The aim of cognitive restructuring is that a more rational and functional thought for these situations are constructed. This process may take a long time, so patients should not expect short-term results.

3.6.6 More Interventions Targeted for Children

While the above interventions can also be used in adolescents with appropriate understanding, there are some known interventions that may already be useful for younger aged children. To minimize scratching, **distraction** with a small toy or game may be useful. Also, the use of **scratching alternatives**, such as cooling of the skin with a "magic stone," may be beneficial. A "**pizza massage**," a massage that follows the same steps as making a pizza, can also be useful in reducing stress or anxiety (see table 3.3)

Table 3.3   How to Do a "Pizza Massage"

1. Knead the dough: squish and press the skin on the child's back lightly

2. Roll out the dough: make gentle rolling motions, either with a wooden massage roller or using your fist, down the back

3. Spread the sauce: make a flat palm and rub it smoothly over the back

4. Add the toppings: ask them what toppings they'd like! Then gently tap and pat the surface of the back

5. Put the pizza in the oven: rub your hands together to create warmth and then place them on the child's back

6. Chop the pizza: use the sides of your hand to gently make chopping motions over the back

Instead of the "pizza-massage," a "**weather massage**" also can be conducted, where the parents pretend that different weather conditions (sunshine, snow, rain, storm . . .) occur.

Habit reversal training (HRT) is an intervention that cannot only be used in adults, but also in children to alter dysfunctional behaviors like hair-pulling or nail-biting. It teaches patients to replace these behaviors with more neutral ones. In the case of chronic itch, this includes replacing scratching as the negative behavior that exacerbates the itch-scratch cycle with neutral behaviors like clenching a fist, holding it for some seconds and then pressing the itchy body site with your nail. Changing this behavior involves three components: raising awareness of the behavior that needs to be replaced (e.g., by describing the scratching and situations that trigger it in great detail), training of the "new" behavior at the first sign of scratching, and motivating yourself to control the habit (e.g., through self-motivation or encouragement from a partner, family member, or therapist). This kind of training has recently been shown to have additional effects to medical treatment in children with atopic dermatitis.

3.6.7 Patient Education Programs

In some countries, patient education programs, also referred to as itch schools or schools for patients with itchy conditions, have been established. These are usually led by a multi-disciplinary team of professionals, including dermatologists, psychologists, nurses, and dieticians. Together, they counsel groups of patients and their families/caregivers on how to manage itchy diseases from their unique perspectives. For example, psychologists may counsel patients on how to react to comments from others regarding their skin, while dieticians may provide information on what foods can aggravate or help to reduce itching. In addition, attending such sessions can provide a sense of community with other patients and improve social support.

Conclusion

Itch is something that affects all of us. For some, it may seem as simple as an annoying mosquito bite that resolves within a few days, but for millions of others, itch can be a persistent, chronic problem that significantly impacts quality of life and overall functioning. While in the past, our incomplete understanding of why this sensation occurs has limited our ability to treat this often-devastating condition, our understanding in recent years has grown tremendously, opening up new frontiers for innovation. Understanding how the mechanisms of itch vary in different conditions has allowed for the discovery of new treatment targets, and clinical trials continue to investigate promising new therapies. While there is no official "cure" for itch, we are closer to eliminating it now than we ever have been before.

Our goal for writing this book was not to provide you with information about a particular disease or treatment option but to show you that you are not alone. There are so many others struggling, searching for answers, and determined to help you on your journey to rid yourself of itch. These include other patients, family members, your doctors and nurses, researchers, psychologists, support groups, and national organizations. In addition, we aimed to showcase the personalized nature of both the itch experience and how to manage it, emphasizing the importance of an individualized and multidisciplinary approach to finding what works best for every individual. We hope that you've learned something new and added to your "anti-itch" toolbox. But most important, we hope that we have given you the understanding and knowledge to maintain hope even on your toughest days. Progress is happening and we look forward to a bright future filled with new treatments for all of our itchy patients!

Resources

General Resource for Patients and Practitioners
International Forum for the Study of Itch: https://www
.itchforum.net

Associations for People with Specific Skin Conditions
The Coalition of Skin Diseases is an umbrella association
composed of member associations that provide education
and support for people with specific skin diseases and disorders. Visit http://www.coalitionofskindiseases.org/ for information about the Coalition of Skin Diseases. Listed below are
other organizations that provide information and support for
people with skin conditions.

Alopecia Areata
National Alopecia Areata Foundation
14 Mitchell Boulevard
San Rafael, CA 94903
Phone (415) 472-3780
E-mail info@naaf.org
www.naaf.org

Basal Cell Carcinoma Nevus Syndrome
Basal Cell Carcinoma Nevus Syndrome (BCCNS Life Support
Network)
PO Box 321, 14525 North Cheshire Street
Burton, OH 44021
Phone (440) 834-0011
E-mail info@bccns.org
www.gorlinsyndrome.org, www.bccns.org

Cicatricial Alopecia
Cicatricial Alopecia Research Foundation (CARF)
9300 Wilshire Boulevard, Suite 410
Beverly Hills, CA 90212
Phone (310) 285-0525
E-mail info@carfintl.org
www.carfintl.org

Cutaneous Lymphoma
Cutaneous Lymphoma Foundation
PO Box 374
Birmingham, MI 48012
Phone (248) 644-9014
E-mail info@CLFoundation.org
www.CLFoundation.org

Ectodermal Dysplasias
National Foundation for Ectodermal Dysplasias (NFED)
6 Executive Drive, Suite 2
Fairview Heights, IL 62208-1360
Phone (618) 566-2020
E-mail info@nfed.org
www.nfed.org

Eczema
National Eczema Association
4460 Redwood Highway, Suite 16D
San Rafael, CA 94903
Phone (415) 499-3474
E-mail info@nationaleczema.org
www.nationaleczema.org

Epidermolysis Bullosa
Debra of America
16 East 41st Street, 3rd Floor
New York, NY 10017
Phone (212) 868-1573
E-mail staff@debra.org
www.debra.org

Ichthyosis
Foundation for Ichthyosis and Related Skin Types
2616 N. Broad Street
Colmar, PA 18915
Phone (215) 997-9400
E-mail info@firstskinfoundation.org
www.firstskinfoundation.org

Large Nevi and Related Disorders
Nevus Outreach, Inc.
600 SE Delaware, Suite 200
Bartlesville, OK 74003
Phone (918) 331-0595
www.nevus.org

Pachyonychia Congenita
Pachyonychia Congenita Project (PC Project)
2386 E. Heritage Way, Suite B
Salt Lake City, UT 84109
Phone (877) 628-7300
E-mail info@pachyonychia.org
www.pachyonychia.org

Pemphigus and Pemphigoid
International Pemphigus and Pemphigoid Foundation (IPPF)
1331 Garden Highway, Suite 100
Sacramento, CA 95833
Phone (916) 922-1298
E-mail info@pemphigus.org
www.pemphigus.org

Prurigo Nodularis
Prurigo Nodularis League
Münster, Germany
http://www.pruritussymposium.de/prurigonodularisleague
.html

Psoriasis
National Psoriasis Foundation
6600 SW 92nd Ave, Suite 300
Portland, OR 97219
Phone (503) 244-7404
E-mail getinfo@psoriasis.org
www.psoriasis.org

Sturge-Weber Syndrome and Klippel-Trenaunay
The Sturge-Weber Foundation
PO Box 418
Mt. Freedom, NJ 07970
Phone (973) 895-4445
E-mail swfl@sturge-weber.com
www.sturge-weber.org

Vitiligo
Vitiligo Support International, Inc. (VSI)
PO Box 3565
Lynchburg, VA 24503
Phone (434) 326-5380
E-mail info@vitiligosupport.org
www.vitiligosupport.org

Xeroderma Pigmentosum
Xeroderma Pigmentosum Family Support Group
8495 Folsom Boulevard #1
Sacramento, CA 95826
Phone (916) 379-0741
E-mail contact@xpfamilysupport.org
www.xpfamilysupport.org

Index

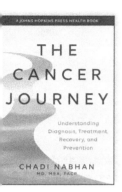

"No matter where along the journey one may be, the book spans the cancer care continuum providing helpful insights and guidance for all."

—Julie Gralow, MD,
Chief Medical Officer, American Society of Clinical Oncology

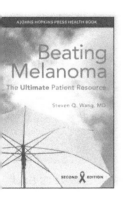

"Dr. Wang's *Beating Melanoma* is the ultimate guide that has woven together the collective wisdom of 25 world medical experts across specialties."

—Deborah Sarnoff,
The Skin Cancer Foundation

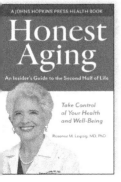

"Essential reading for anyone who is growing older or whose loved ones are growing older."

—Martha Stewart

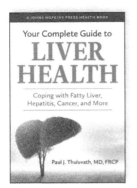

"Dr. Thuluvath provides in a layperson's language the framework by which physicians diagnose, stage, and manage liver diseases."

—Joseph K. Lim, MD,
Yale University School of Medicine

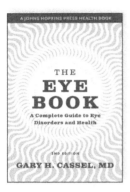

"This guide covers routine eyecare and the more common eye diseases, providing up-to-date facts on refractive surgery, treatment for optical neuritis, and possible nutritional therapies for cataracts and macular degeneration."

—*Library Journal*

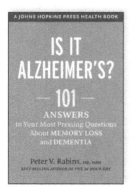

"*Is It Alzheimer's?* offers honest answers and positive bottom-line approaches to tough decisions and questions."

—Lisa P. Gwyther,
Founder, Duke Dementia Family Support Program

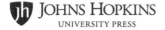 JOHNS HOPKINS UNIVERSITY PRESS | PRESS.JHU.EDU |